CANNABIS BRITANNICA

Empire, Trade, and Prohibition
1800–1928

JAMES H. MILLS

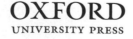
OXFORD
UNIVERSITY PRESS

OXFORD
UNIVERSITY PRESS

Great Clarendon Street, Oxford OX2 6DP

Oxford University Press is a department of the University of Oxford.
It furthers the University's objective of excellence in research, scholarship,
and education by publishing worldwide in

Oxford New York

Auckland Bangkok Buenos Aires Cape Town Chennai
Dar es Salaam Delhi Hong Kong Istanbul Karachi Kolkata
Kuala Lumpur Madrid Melbourne Mexico City Mumbai Nairobi
São Paulo Shanghai Taipei Tokyo Toronto

Oxford is a registered trade mark of Oxford University Press
in the UK and in certain other countries

Published in the United States
by Oxford University Press Inc., New York

© James H. Mills 2003

The moral rights of the author have been asserted
Database right Oxford University Press (maker)

First published 2003

British Library Cataloguing in Publication Data
Data available

Library of Congress Cataloging in Publication Data
Data available

ISBN 0–19–924938–5

1 3 5 7 9 10 8 6 4 2

Typeset by Kolam Information Services Pvt. Ltd. Pondicherry, India
Printed in Great Britain on acid-free paper by
T.J. International Ltd, Padstow, Cornwall

For my loves, Rebecca and Constance

Preface

The debate about cannabis and the law in the media, in government circles, and in the scientific and medical communities will continue to intensify. Recent changes in policy, contested experiments with tolerant policing, and the forthcoming release of results from UK medical trials form the background to the ongoing controversies about the extent to which cannabis substances ought to be regulated by the law and how far they are properly the concern of government agencies and of politicians.

For all this debate and all these controversies it is a curious fact that the origins of Britain's current laws and of government policies on cannabis remain unknown. After all, if the regulations and positions currently adhered to were put in place for sound and rational reasons then this would considerably bolster the position of those who advocate continuity. On the other hand, if these restrictions and approaches were the outcome of poor research or hidden agendas then the argument of those who demand change would be strengthened. History would seem to have a key place in current debates and to promise fresh perspectives.

This book therefore begins the task of examining the historical origins of Britain's laws and policies on cannabis. The approach is to determine what information was available in any given period and the extent to which officials, administrators, and legislators referred to that knowledge or were guided by other factors in reaching their decisions. The book covers the period to 1928 when the Coca Leaves and Indian Hemp Regulations found cannabis its own place in British law for the first time. A second, forthcoming volume will examine the period from 1928 to the present day.

A large number of people are owed a debt for their help in the completion of this book. The sources used are from a number of countries and a range of archives and so my thanks are due to staff in the National Archives of India in Delhi, the Maharashtra State Archives in Mumbai, the Agra Mental Hospital, the British Library (in particular the India Office Library and the Rare Books rooms), the Wellcome Trust Library, the Public Record Office, the National Library of Scotland, and Edinburgh University Library. Financial assistance for this work was given by the Carnegie Trust for the Universities of Scotland, the Wellcome Trust, and above all the ESRC and I am grateful to each for having the imagination to fund work in this area.

A range of academics and professionals also played a part in the development of this book. Dr Crispin Bates in the Department of History at Edinburgh University offered, as usual, a number of perceptive remarks on my work and Professor Pete King at UCN was unfailingly supportive in many aspects of my research. Professor Virginia Berridge and Dr Sarah Mars at the London School of Hygiene and Tropical Medicine provided interesting comments on the twentieth-century material. Dr Aditya Kumar of the Agra Mental Hospital allowed me access to the set of nineteenth-century psychiatric case notes that are in his personal collection and Drs Sanjeev Jain and Pratima Murthy invited me to use the rich set of sources available at the National Institute of Mental Health and Neurological Sciences in Bangalore. Dr Satadru Sen of Washington University, St Louis, was an excellent sounding board during a research trip to Delhi in 1999. My thanks go to them all.

While researching and writing this book I also managed to marry Rebecca and between us we started a family with the birth of our daughter, Constance Verity. All of my work is for them, with love.

Contents

A Note on Terms

The following definitions are taken from the *Report of the Indian Hemp Drugs Commission* (Simla, 1894), i. 59.

Ganja consists of the dried flowering tops of cultivated female hemp plants which have become coated with resin in consequence of having been unable to set seeds freely.

Charas [and hashish] is the name applied to the resinous matter which forms the active principle when collected separately.

Siddhi, bhang, subzi or patti are different names applied to the dry leaves of the hemp plant, whether male or female, and whether cultivated or uncultivated.

These definitions have been generally accepted by the witnesses but the result of the inquiries is to show that they require some explanation. First with regard to ganja.

Over nearly the whole of India distinction is recognised between the ganja and the bhang plant. Though the natives may mistake the sexes, it is clear that the female plant is the one called ganja and the male plant bhang. The plants are distinguishable even in the wild state, the loose flowering panicle of the male from the comparatively stiff and apparently bottomless spike of the female. The hill ganja of Assam and the wild ganja that seems to be occasionally found and used throughout Eastern Bengal and the sub-Himalayan region and even in Kashmir must be the female flower spike which has often been quite innocent of any tending. In examining the evidence therefore the definition of ganja given above must often be read as with the word cultivated omitted.

Then as regards bhang the witnesses often use the word to include the female flower head as well as the leaves of the plant and the green leaves as well as the dry. The male flower head must also enter into it in consequence of the rude method of preparing the drug viz. by drying the plants and beating out the leaves. But the male flowers are not more narcotic than the leaves; the point to be noted is the inclusion of the female flower head in bhang. The confusion arises from the name of the product bhang being used also for the liquid form in which the hemp drugs are consumed. Ganja pounded up and made into drink becomes bhang. This is the way in which Garhjat ganja is used in Puri. In the west and south of India the distinction between the products bhang and ganja is frequently lost. Bhang is cultivated in Sind with similar precautions to prevent the fertilization of the female plant as in Bengal and the product is called nothing but bhang and is rarely used for anything but concocting drink and sweetmeats, the smoking ganja being imported. Bhang is the ancient name of the plant. It is also the name of the form of narcotic product which was earliest discovered for it must have taken time to learn the art of isolating the female plant and so producing ganja. Bhang is also the name of the most simple style of consumption, viz., by pounding and drinking which must have preceded smoking. Naturally, therefore, bhang is a more comprehensive term than ganja and often includes it, especially where the production of ganja has not become a recognised industry. In the Madras Presidency ganja is the more general term so much so that in some places the word bhang is hardly understood. This is probably due to the hemp plant being only known to the people as cultivated for production of ganja.

Charas may not always be the pure resinous matter. It generally contains leaf dust and other impurities picked up in the process of manufacture. But it is hardly ever confounded with ganja or bhang. Its appearance, that of dark green or brown paste, is distinct from that of both the other drugs. In Kashmir and the Punjab only is the name ganja sometimes applied to charas, probably because charas is prepared from the female organja plant (Governor of Kashmir). There is reason to think that in some parts of Rajputana the distinction between charas and ganja is not very strictly observed, and that the former name is occasionally given to the latter drug.

List of Illustrations

between pp. 116–117

1. Gouache by an Amritsar artist depicting the smoking of Charras, a type of Indian hemp imported into northern India from Eastern Turkestan. Archaeological Survey of India Collections: India Office Series (Volume 49). The painting accompanied samples of the narcotics illustrated, and was made for display at an unidentified exhibition. India Office Photograph 1000/49(4782). Copyright © The British Library Board.

2. Gouache by an Amritsar artist depicting the preparation and consumption of Indian hemp (bhang). Archaeological Survey of India Collections: India Office Series (Volume 49). The painting accompanied samples of the narcotics illustrated, and was made for display at an unidentified exhibition. India Office Photograph 1000/49 (4783). Copyright © The British Library Board.

3. Bhang. Anonymous, opaque watercolour *c*.1850, Rajasthan/Jaipur style. India Office Drawing Add.Or.2835. Copyright © The British Library Board.

4. Men preparing and smoking Indian hemp. Anonymous watercolour *c*.1860, Punjab style. India Office Drawing Add.Or.1451. Copyright © The British Library Board.

5. A zemindar. Goojur landholder. Saharunpoor *c*.1860s. J. Forbes Watson and John William Kaye, *The People of India. A Series of Photographic Illustrations, with Descriptive Letterpress, of the Races and Tribes of Hindustan*, Volume III (India Museum, London, 1868). India Office Photo 973/3(157). Copyright © The British Library Board.

6. A nineteenth-century sketch of the female cannabis plant in India. R. Wissett, *A Treatise on Hemp*, (London 1808). 434h.19 Copyright © The British Library Board.

7. Portrait of the Reverend Thomas Evans. Evans was William Caine's companion on the latter's tour of India in 1889. He was also a committed temperance campaigner and a harsh critic of cannabis intoxicants in India. D. Hooper (ed.), *A Welshman in India: A Record of the Life of Thomas Evans, Missionary* (London, 1908). National Library of Scotland.

8. Portrait of William Sproston Caine MP. Caine mounted a one-man campaign against the Government of India on the issue of cannabis substances and secured the Indian Hemp Drugs Commission of 1893/4. J. Newton, *W.S. Caine, M.P.: A Biography* (London, 1907). National Library of Scotland.

9. Frontpage of the Report of the Indian Hemp Drugs Commission of 1894. This is the most extensive survey of a cannabis-using society by a Western government to date. National Library of Scotland.

10. Group of Gossavis, habitual excessive ganja smokers, Khandesh. This photograph was taken for, and included in, the Report of the Indian Hemp Drugs Commission of 1894. It was one of a series depicting cannabis users who were grouped according to the frequency of use of the drug. National Library of Scotland.

1

Introduction

THE STORY OF CANNABIS AND BRITISH GOVERNMENT

It has been formerly believed to render Persons unactive in Venereal
Affairs; but that is not at all likely, for it not only causes Hens to lay
Eggs in Plenty, if given moderately; but the famous Bangue so much
used by Persians and Indians to promote Venery, is a Species of Hemp.

R. James, *A Medicinal Dictionary*, 1745.[1]

The Hemp plant has been cultivated in Bengal from time immemorial
for the purpose of intoxication; but is never used by the natives for
cordage or cloth as in Europe. The plant is called by them *ganja* and
the intoxicating preparation made from it *Bang*.

R. Wissett, *On the Cultivation and Preparation of Hemp*, 1804.[2]

I am certain that you gentlemen who work under the aegis of the
League of Nations, will help us in the struggle we have undertaken
against this scourge which reduces man to the level of the brute and
deprives him of health and reason, self-control and honour.

Mohammed El Guindy, *Speech to the Second Opium
Conference*, 1924.[3]

Although cannabis substances experienced only periodic popularity as
medicines and were little used as recreational drugs in the United Kingdom

---

[1] R. James, *A Medicinal Dictionary, including Physic, Surgery, Anatomy, Chymistry and Botany in all
their branches relative to medicine together with a history of drugs, an account of their various preparations,
combinations, and uses* (Osborne, London, 1745).

[2] R. Wissett, *On the Cultivation and Preparation of Hemp* (Cox & Son, London, 1804), 18.

[3] *Records of the Second Opium Conference*, vol. i (12 Dec. 1924), 135.

before the 1950s, the above quotes suggest that the British, their governments, and Indian hemp products have enjoyed a long and colourful history. In the eighteenth century cannabis preparations were the subject of prurient curiosity in the medical and scientific circles of London where they were regarded as one of the more exotic and mysterious of the exciting new drugs and medicines coming on to the home market from Britain's imperial possessions and mercantile outposts. By the early nineteenth century, however, the cannabis sativa plant was a major concern for British governments. They were little interested in its intoxicating properties and far more enthusiastic about its potential as a source of cordage for the rigging of the navy upon which the security of the nation and the exploitation of the empire depended. By the twentieth century cannabis substances were occupying the time of Britain's diplomats, as they sought to protect the lucrative imperial income from the cannabis trade of India from the determined lobbying of countries who wanted to impose international laws on the world's drugs supplies.

Of course, these quotes can only convey three parts of a far more complex story. This book will examine all of the key figures and events in the modern history of cannabis and British government. The story starts in Chapter 2, which shows how information about cannabis drugs and medicines was slowly gathered in Asia by Europeans from the sixteenth century onwards. The men responsible for this were the Iberian doctors that accompanied the Portuguese empire-builders into India and their observations, together with those of the ancient authorities like Dioscorides, remained the basis of British writing on the subject of cannabis into the eighteenth century. In that century accounts of cannabis were embellished by British travellers returning from Asia who were eager to sell their stories of journeys abroad by filling them with lurid tales of exotic vices. It was not until the nineteenth century that scientists and doctors serving in the empire began to turn their systematic attention to the subject. While some viewed cannabis medicines and drugs through their own prejudices others seemed to have been determined to light up the subject with the full glare of Victorian science. Of the latter, perhaps William Brooke O'Shaughnessy was the most thorough and the most remarkable. The man who is often credited with saving the British Empire in India in the 1850s conducted a range of experiments with cannabis in the 1830s in Calcutta, where he served as Professor of Chemistry and Medicine in the Medical College. Dogs, cats, pigs, goats, crows, vultures, and even fish were observed while under the influence of cannabis and eventually his patients and his students were dosed with preparations of the plant and their responses were carefully recorded. Among the conditions that he treated with the medicine were rheumatism, rabies, tetanus, and cholera. By 1839 he was sufficiently confident to conclude that 'the results seem to me to warrant our anticipating from its more extensive and impartial use no inconsiderable addition to the resources of the physician'. Once back in England he presented his results to an enthusiastic meeting of the Royal Medico-Botanical Society that heralded the arrival of cannabis in the box of remedies resorted to by the nineteenth-century British doctor.

Chapter 3 returns to India and considers the other side of British interest in cannabis. While scientists of the empire like O'Shaughnessy were investigating hemp drugs for their medical benefits his colleagues in the East India Company revenue offices were sizing them up for their financial potential. The British in India, who made such vast profits as the world's largest peddlers of opium to China, taxed the cannabis trade. They did this because, in India, they found themselves in control of the world's largest market for and trade in cannabis drugs. These were produced locally and consumed across the region's classes, castes, and religions as medicines, tonics, and intoxicants. As they were in Asia primarily for economic gain it quickly occurred to British officials to cream off a revenue by way of levying a tax on the commerce in cannabis and they began to do this as early as the 1790s. The records of the excise officers remain a rich source for exploring a society where use of cannabis products was well established and extensive and for examining the ways in which British administrators viewed the drug and formulated strategies for taxing trade in it. However, as they controlled such a booming cannabis economy and sought to profit from it these administrators encountered producers determined to evade taxation and smugglers eager to carry contraband to the market-place. The British, who had fought wars and extended their Indian territories to secure their profits from opium drugs in Asia, were equally set on guaranteeing their income from cannabis. As such, they began to impose increasingly complex customs systems and to advocate harsher systems of surveillance on cannabis producing regions, and to view as criminals those producers who sought to guarantee their profit margins by evading the law. It is in this period in India, and because of this determination of the Raj to seize a revenue from the commerce in cannabis, that the plant and its preparations first began to be associated with criminality in the minds of British government officials.

Chapter 4 shows that while many British doctors and scientists continued to view cannabis as a useful medicine throughout the nineteenth century others were expressing serious doubts about its impact on the human mind. While debate occurred in the medical press of the UK it was from India that the most compelling evidence of a relationship between cannabis use and insanity was being produced by British medical officers. Statistics compiled at the lunatic asylums of colonial India seemed to show that a significant proportion of the cases treated were caused by use of cannabis preparations. By the 1870s these statistics had sparked a colony-wide inquiry by the Government of India that was eager to locate sources of disorder in the society that it was trying to control. The inquiry concluded that habitual use of cannabis substances tended to produce insanity and was the first time that a British administration gave an official verdict on cannabis. The problem, however, is that the statistics on which this verdict was based were severely flawed. The rest of the chapter discusses why this was the case and shows that the Victorians themselves later realized this. However, by the time they did, the statistics had been so widely accepted as scientific evidence of the link between mental illness and use of cannabis that few revised their opinion.

Indeed, by the 1890s these statistics from the lunatic asylums of India had become an issue back in Britain and in the House of Commons itself. A Scottish temperance campaigner, Mark Stewart MP, called the attention of the House of Commons in 1891 to a report that the lunatic asylums of India were filled with ganja smokers. William Sproston Caine, the heir to a Cheshire iron ore fortune and MP for Bradford, took up the case and demanded an inquiry into the profits made by the British in India from trade in cannabis products. This sudden parliamentary interest in the 1890s does not reflect an innate concern about cannabis itself but rather shows how the subject became entangled in the broader controversies of the period. Veteran anti-opium campaigners, temperance advocates, and bitter critics of imperialism allied to use the issue of Britain's drugs profits in Asia in order to question the nature of both Gladstone's government and of the Raj itself. Vehemently opposed to Britain's position as the world's largest organized supplier of narcotics, these critics saw cannabis as yet another stick with which to beat the administration. As such it suited them to portray hemp as 'the most horrible intoxicant the world has yet produced' once they had discovered that the colonial authorities in India derived a revenue from it. Yet having succeeded in forcing the government to establish the Indian Hemp Drugs Commission (IHDC) to investigate the issue the campaigners quickly lost interest in the subject. This was largely because the Commission concluded that cannabis was certainly not the world's most horrible intoxicant. Compiled by both British officials and Indian notables, the eight volumes of the IHDC's report remains one of the most complete surveys of a cannabis consuming society to this day. It denied any link between social problems and cannabis use and indeed claimed that 'moderate' and 'habitual' use of cannabis had no health implications and that only 'excessive' use was to be avoided. It also argued strenuously that the asylum statistics that had been used to give scientific weight to the argument that cannabis use caused mental illness were unreliable enough to be dismissed. But the IHDC is not above suspicion when it comes to political agendas as two of the three Indian delegates refused to sign the final report, feeling that it had ignored important evidence in its eagerness to absolve cannabis use in India, and the revenue that the colonial government derived from it, from troubling associations. Chapter 5 investigates the place of cannabis in the broader drugs politics of the 1890s and looks at the question of how the British came to conduct one of the most important inquiries into cannabis of modern history.

Chapter 6, in contrast, explores the period after the IHDC when cannabis dropped off the political agenda. Indians continued to consume large quantities of cannabis and the British administration continued to cream off an income through taxation from suppliers of this market. It was in the bastions of British medicine and science, rather than in those of politics and government, that interest in hemp substances flourished in the period 1894–1912. The complaint by British doctors since the time of W. B. O'Shaughnessy had been that while cannabis medicines might be useful it was difficult to secure a supply of reliable raw materials from which to make medicinal concoctions. Because the potency of each batch was variable it was difficult to produce medicines that were consistent in strength and predictable in outcome and so the race was on to locate the active ingredient. From 1897 onwards it was British scientists that led the way in London and at Cambridge. Wood, Spivey, and Easterfield pioneered research in this period—indeed Spivey was to die mysteriously in experiments with oxy-cannabin—and they located a toxic red oil or resin from cannabis in 1897 and called it 'cannabinol'. C. R Marshall, who went on to become Professor of Materia Medica and Therapeutics at St Andrews University continued trials of this cannabinol over the next decade as did W. E. Dixon at St Thomas's Hospital in London. He was so impressed by the potential of cannabis that he continued to advocate it throughout an illustrious career in which he became Reader in Pharmacology at Cambridge and a member of the Rolleston Committee on Morphine and Heroin Addiction in 1925. Experiments in the scientific community meanwhile were mirrored in creative circles, where there is evidence that Bohemian elements took to 'hashish' in order to

explore consciousness. However, the drug remained known only to
scientists, doctors, and to this tiny clique among the nation's artistic elite
and the population as a whole had no awareness of cannabis and its
properties.

Despite the fact that cannabis remained largely unknown by the majority
of the British population, preparations of the substance became the subject
of UK legislation for the first time in the 1920s. Chapters 7 and 8 examine
the reasons for this. The former concentrates on the international scene and
looks at the political clouds that gathered over the British position in global
systems of drugs supply. As the world's chief supplier of opium to Chinese
markets the British administration in India became the subject of both
domestic and international condemnation that continued into the twentieth
century. Indeed, once the Americans adopted a holier-than-thou attitude
towards opium consumption in their own colonies they began to construct
a diplomatic platform from which to foist international controls on drugs
supply between countries. This evolved into the League of Nations Advisory Council on Opium after the First World War and led to the two
opium conferences of 1924–5. While the focus of these agencies was
opium, and to a lesser extent cocaine, cannabis exploded on to the agenda
at the Second Opium Conference in 1924.

Egypt was a country like India where 'hashish' was used extensively as a
medicine, as a tonic, and as an intoxicant. However, its government was
emerging from the colonial rule of the British and was eager to be seen to be
reformist. As such its delegation stood at the Second Opium Conference
to insist that their government's attempts to control cannabis consumption
among the Egyptian population were being hampered by an international
trade in the substance that allowed smugglers to secure supplies to sell
in their country. The Egyptians wanted trade in the drug to be outlawed
and the rest of the delegates, who knew nothing of cannabis and who were
there to argue about opium, seemed to be ready to agree to the demand. It
was left to the British, who still drew a considerable revenue from the drugs
in India, to resist the radical proposals of the Egyptians. Sir Malcolm
Delevingne of the Home Office, a career bureaucrat and one of the pioneers
of British drug policy, employed all of his diplomatic wiles to distract the
meeting from Egypt's agenda. Nevertheless the African delegation, egged
on by American support, succeeded in forcing a watered-down version of
their demands into the final agreement of the Conference. Obliged to ratify
this because they were a member of the League of Nations, the British
ended up with regulations on cannabis that their diplomats had opposed.
The irony of all this was that it may well have been British colonial officials

working in Egypt that gave the Egyptian delegates their ammunition for the Conference in the first place.

By the time the agreement of the Second Opium Conference was incorporated into British law by the Coca Leaves and Indian Hemp Regulations of 1928 another set of restrictions had already been imposed upon cannabis. In 1924 the Pharmaceutical Society elected to include cannabis in the Poisons Schedule, thereby imposing a set of controls on who could buy and sell cannabis substances. It explained that it had taken this step because of recent cases where cannabis had come before the courts. Cannabis substances had briefly enjoyed a flurry of media attention as the result of arrests made in London. Two Africans, one a war veteran and both waiters in coffee shops in the West End of London, had been apprehended by detectives on a charge of attempting to supply opium. Once the policemen discovered that the substance offered by the two dealers was in fact 'hashish' they pretended that they had known this all along and began to lobby the Home Office to include cannabis in the Dangerous Drugs Act. At the time there were no restrictions on the possession or supply of cannabis substances and the police ended up looking rather silly as the case against the two men was thrown out of court. The newspapers, however, found the story thrilling as it combined West End locations, exotic immigrants, and mysterious drugs. Despite media attention and police lobbying, the Home Office utterly refused to countenance the addition of cannabis to existing laws. It investigated a number of odd cases involving cannabis in the 1920s, including traces of the drug in cigarette tobacco in Shrewsbury and lumps of the substance hidden in a coal shed on Tyneside, and concluded that cannabis was little used and certainly not implicated in any problems of law and social order. Indeed, medical and scientific experts continued to debate the merits of the substance and powerful advocates spoke in its defence. However, it seems that the Pharmaceutical Society, which alone had the power to classify substances as poisons, ignored the Home Office and the experts and instead was panicked by police bungling and media hype. Chapter 8 examines this domestic history of cannabis regulation and shows how policy seems to have been driven by mistakes and misunderstandings rather than by well-informed debate.

The book taken as a whole then tells the first part of the history of the British, their governments, and cannabis drugs in the modern period and looks at how the country first came in the 1920s to have restrictions that dealt specifically with those substances. The second half of the story will come in a subsequent volume.

HISTORY, CANNABIS, AND CURRENT DEBATES

This book, however, is not simply a whimsical tale from faraway places and long ago times. It may be directly relevant to contemporary debates about laws and polices relating to cannabis in Britain today. This is because politicians continue to this day to turn to the past in order to defend, or sometimes to challenge, current positions on cannabis. For example, as recently as 1999 the government rejected the Select Committee on Science and Technology's recommendations that cannabinol be reclassified in Schedule 2 of the Misuse of Drugs Act in order to allow doctors to prescribe it for medical use. In doing this, the government claimed that it had a 'firmly grounded and logical position on the availability of cannabis for therapeutic purposes'.[4] This position was that cannabis was in Schedule 1 of the Misuse of Drugs Regulations that listed 'those substances which are not generally acknowledged to have therapeutic value'. For it to be moved to Schedule 2 it would be necessary for advocates of cannabis to demonstrate its 'safety, quality and efficacy', as indeed is the case for all other prospective medicines. This defence rested on a historical assumption, that is that cannabinol had been correctly scheduled in the first place.

However, a consideration of the period in the early 1970s when cannabis substances were originally scheduled is revealing, as it seems that history was again central to the reasoning of those in government. The MPs drafting the 1971 Misuse of Drugs Act appear to have simply pointed to the status quo in considering calls for change.

The present Government, like the previous Government, have no option but to deal with cannabis in as zealous a light as was the case for many years previously. Until and unless there is clear evidence to the contrary there would be no justification for acting differently.[5]

It seems then that the Blair government has defended its policy using the assumption that its predecessors had good reasons for arriving at their assessments of cannabis and that their judgements were based on solid ground. However, it seems that their predecessors were content not to dig too deeply into the issue and had themselves simply advocated continuity with the past. It appears then that there is in fact a history of history being used to defend cannabis policy, but in both instances a search through the

---

[4] Select Committee on Science and Technology 2nd Report 1998–9, *Cannabis: Government Response* (The Stationery Office, London, 1999), 7.
[5] Standing Committee A, *Misuse of Drugs Bill*, 17 Nov. 1970, p. 229.

documents that accompany these references to the past suggests that there was no actual knowledge of what that past was.

However, history has not simply been used to defend cannabis policy. Consider the argument of the Select Committee on Science and Technology in 1999 in criticizing the present government's stance.

Both the Medicines Control Agency and the Home Office persist in treating cannabis-based medicines as new medicines. Cannabis, however, has a history of medical use in man stretching back hundreds of years. For much of the nineteenth century and the first half of the twentieth century, moreover, it was administered in Britain as a tincture (cannabis oil in alcohol); thus the oral administration of cannabis extracts which contain significant quantities of cannabidiol has a long history of medicinal use. In choosing to ignore the long history of safe therapeutic cannabis use, and in classifying cannabis extract (and cannabidiol) as a 'new medicine' the Government and the MCA are treating a long-established herbal extract as if it were just another new synthetic chemical, and are thus not making an informed scientific judgement.[6]

The Select Committee does at least demonstrate in this statement that it has taken the trouble to establish a few facts. However, the problem with this statement is that there are many examples from the past that can be used to refute it. Plenty of stories can be found in the archives that suggest that cannabis was not always safely used as a therapy and indeed that suggest that intoxication rather than treatment was sometimes the reason for its consumption. Quite simply, in this case a few facts are almost as useless as no facts at all, as the partial account provided gives only a glimpse of the overall picture. There are those in government then that defend current positions on cannabis by reference to the past and there are also those that would challenge these positions with such historical references. The problem is that on both sides there is a dearth of wide-ranging, detailed, and accurate knowledge.

That the government lacks this knowledge of the origins of current laws and policies is no great surprise given the fact that most of the information on cannabis with which they are confronted fails to concern itself with historical issues. Official institutional surveys are especially guilty of this. The British Medical Association for example published its report in 1997 on *Therapeutic Uses of Cannabis*.[7] It recommended that 'the Government should consider changing the Misuse of Drugs Act to allow the

[6] Select Committee on Science and Technology, 2nd Report 2000–1, *Therapeutic Uses of Cannabis* (www.parliament.the-stationery-office.co.uk).

[7] British Medical Association, *Therapeutic Uses of Cannabis* (Harwood Academic Publishers, Amsterdam, 1997).

prescription of cannabinoids to patients with particular medical conditions that are not adequately controlled by existing treatments'.[8] It also urged that 'police, the courts and other prosecuting authorities should be aware of the medicinal reasons for the unlawful use of cannabis by those suffering from certain medical conditions'.[9] In other words it advocated changes in existing laws and indeed in existing attitudes by a range of official bodies including the government, the police, the judiciary, and the magistracy. It suggested these changes, however, for purely medical and scientific reasons, and although it did not see cannabis itself as a useful medicine, it had been satisfied after its review of the evidence that certain cannabinoids present in cannabis 'are remarkably safe drugs with a side-effects profile superior to many drugs used for the same indications'.[10] It did note briefly that 'in this country, the medicinal use of cannabis was particularly prominent in the nineteenth century. However it remained permissible for British doctors to prescribe cannabis (as a tincture for oral administration) until 1971.'[11] On the whole, however, the report was uninterested in the history of the laws and attitudes that it sought to change and was solely concerned with scientific arguments. A similar document by the Academy of Medical Sciences that also focused on scientific data forwarded exactly the opposite recommendation, namely that 'there is no persuasive case for the non-experimental medical use of cannabis'. While acknowledging that there is plenty of anecdotal evidence both for the benefits of cannabis medicines and for their harmful side effects, it reached its conclusion simply because there was insufficient clinical trial data on which to base a recommendation for change.[12]

Information-based charity Drugscope published its survey of the cannabis issue in 1998. The report made no recommendations but did contain some useful historical data. It noted that cannabis has a long record of use as a herb and intoxicant, that it was used in 'Parisian salons' in the nineteenth century, that it was favoured by Queen Victoria's physician, that the British had conducted the Indian Hemp Drugs Commission back in 1893–4, and that it was popular in jazz clubs and among 'immigrant groups' in the twentieth century. The problem with such a list is that it is exactly that, simply a list of intriguing facts that are not explained, analysed,

[8] British Medical Association, *Therapeutic Uses of Cannabis* (Hardwood Academic Publishers, Amsterdam, 1997), 78.
   [9] Ibid. 81.   [10] Ibid. 78.   [11] Ibid. 3.
   [12] Academy of Medical Sciences, *The Use of Cannabis and its Derivatives for Medical and Recreational Purposes* (The Royal Society, London, 1998), 3.

or related to one another. On the issue of British laws it did make an important observation:

In Britain, personal use of cannabis was first prohibited in 1928, after an impassioned denunciation by the chief Egyptian delegate persuaded an international opium conference to include it in a list of banned substances.[13]

However, the report did not take this statement any further and, as with the other facts offered, the lack of explanation leaves the reader with more questions than answers. The issues of whether this was a good or a bad decision, whether it was a rational or irrational policy, whether it was a well-considered or ill-judged moment, and so on are left unaddressed.

If official institutional reports offer little by way of history then there are other sources available. Sadly, these also neglect to provide complete or comprehensive accounts of the history of British cannabis laws and policies. Indeed, many of the books that deal with cannabis fail even to rouse a cursory interest in these topics, preferring on the whole to amuse readers with vague assertions about the long-distant past. Such accounts generally refer to a variety of myths and palaeo-botanical guesses to speculate as to whether cannabis may or may not in fact be native to Central Asia, they lavish attention on its use in the ancient urban cultures of China, Scythia, and India, and they guess that it was spread round the world at first by Arab seafarers and subsequently by European ones. Some of these accounts make it past the ancient period and retell the old medieval myth about the assassins, an Islamic sect whose warriors were supposed to have been inspired to fight by use of cannabis drugs. There are even those books that make it past this fine old story to trace evidence of a more general use of the drugs in medieval societies.[14] More useful than such volumes is Virginia Berridge's *Opium and the People* and the number of recent books that trace the development of the international policing of drugs. Berridge focuses

[13] G. Hayes and H. Shapiro, *Drug Notes: Cannabis* (Institute for the Study of Drug Dependence, London, 1998), 13.

[14] M. Merlin, *Man and Marijuana: Some Aspects of their Ancient Relationship* (Associated University Presses, Rutherford, NS, 1972), 24–6; E. Abel, *Marihuana: The First Twelve Thousand Years* (Plenum Press, London, 1980), 4–5, 36–60, 76–104; D. Courtwright, *Forces of Habit: drugs and the Making of the Modern World* (Harvard University Press, London, 2001), 39–41; Brian du Toit, 'Dagga: The History and Ethnographic Setting of Cannabis Sativa in Southern Africa', in V. Rubin (ed.), *Cannabis and Culture* (Mouton, Paris, 1975), 81–116; M. Jay, *Emperors of Dreams: Drugs in the Nineteenth Century* (Dedalus, Sawtry, 2000), 92–5; for a challenge to the old myth of the 'assassins' see L. Iversen, *The Science of Marijuana* (Oxford University Press, Oxford, 2000), 21–2; S. Benet, 'Early Diffusion and Folk Uses of Hemp' and A. Khalifa, 'Traditional Patterns of Hashish Use in Egypt', in Rubin, *Cannabis and Culture*, 39–50 and 195–206; G. Chaturvedi et al., 'Medicinal Use of Opium and Cannabis in Medieval India', *Indian Journal of History of Science* 16/1 (1981), 31–5.

largely on the social history of opium and of opium policy in the UK, but
she does briefly consider cannabis substances and offers the useful conclusions that in the nineteenth-century period 'there was no perceived problem
of domestic cannabis use' and in the twentieth century 'cannabis was
included in the 1925 [Geneva] convention at the request of the Egyptians'.[15] It is the political rather than the social history of opium that is the
concern of Emdad-ul Haq's authoritative account of the development of the
trade in narcotics in South Asia. He does, however, mention cannabis
substances in the nineteenth century and identifies the fact that during this
period 'the [British colonial] government maintained a monopoly system in
cannabis production in north Bengal'.[16] William McAllister's *Drug Diplomacy in the Twentieth Century* is useful for identifying developments such as
the moment that the Italians suggested that cannabis substances were a
matter for the consideration of the Hague Opium Conference in 1911, the
first time that they were introduced into the deliberations of the emerging
international debate on drugs.[17] Taken together then, these accounts offer
important clues as to the diverse origins of British cannabis laws and
policies but none of the volumes does more than mention cannabis in
passing, and where relevant to their other concerns.

Of the popular books available on cannabis in the modern period the
most recent are nothing more than journalistic reportage. Stuart Walton,
who calls himself a wine critic, seems more interested in flaunting his West
End cool by recounting tales 'of patrons of a social club just off Charing
Cross Road [who] were able, until a risibly overdone police swoop in 1998
put a stop to it, to buy bags of high-grade hydroponic skunk from a cashier at
a hatchway on the top floor' than in finding out why the authorities had the
power to make such a raid in the first place.[18] Patrick Matthews, another
self-styled wine writer, published *Cannabis Culture: A Journey through
Disputed Territory* in 1999. This was written as a travelogue through selected

[15] V. Berridge, *Opium and the People* (Free Association Books, London, 1999), 209–15 and
280–2.

[16] M. Emdad-ul Haq, *Drugs in South Asia: From the Opium Trade to the Present Day* (Palgrave,
London, 2000), 33; readers interested in the historical issues raised by Emdad-ul Haq should also see
A. Farooqui, *Smuggling as Subversion: Colonialism, Indian Merchants and the Politics of Opium* (New
Age, New Delhi, 1998).

[17] W. McAllister, *Drug Diplomacy in the Twentieth Century* (Routledge, London, 2000), 31; other
recent books that are useful for tracing the development of the drugs trade and the international
system of control are K. Meyer and T. Parssinen, *Webs of Smoke* (Rowan & Littlefield, London,
1998), and W. Walker, *Opium and Foreign Policy: The Anglo-American Search for Order in Asia,
1912–1954* (University of North Carolina Press, Durham, NC, 1991).

[18] S. Walton, *Out of It: A Cultural History of Intoxication* (Hamish Hamilton, London, 2001),
95–100.

parts of the world cannabis trade, in which he entertained himself by attending trials of those caught in possession of cannabis in Britain and by following meetings of those that campaigned for its legalization. He does offer a history of cannabis and the British that begins to point in the right direction. However, his brief account of colonial experiences of the drug, of attention to the issue in the 1890s, and of the Geneva Opium Conference of 1924–5 is too general to be genuinely informative and he quickly moves attention on to what he finds much more interesting, that is the pro-cannabis campaigners' conspiracy theories.[19]

This focus on conspiracy theories reflects the domination of the literature on cannabis in the modern period by the American story. Writers on cannabis laws and policies in the United States certainly do not suffer from the dearth of detail or the lack of interest in the past that seem to afflict their British colleagues. The favourite conspiracy theory argues that the industrial giant DuPont campaigned in the USA in the 1930s to have production of the cannabis plant heavily taxed and regulated. It did this because the company's business in oil, coal, and wood pulp was threatened by techno-logical advances that meant that hemp would become a rival source of energy and paper. The result of this campaign by DuPont was the 1937 Marihuana Tax Act that stipulated that all importers, manufacturers, sellers, and distributors of hemp had to register with the Secretary of the Treasury and pay an 'occupational tax' on their dealings in the plant. The conspiracy theorists point out that the burden of these taxes killed the hemp industry in America and also acted to deny Americans access to the bene-fits of consuming preparations of the plant.[20]

The evidence for this conspiracy theory is very limited indeed. Other historians prefer to tell another story that has rather more factual support. An energetic American government official, Harry Anslinger, was fresh from his failure as Assistant Commissioner of Prohibition when he was appointed head of the new Bureau of Narcotics in 1930. A professional bureaucrat, he now found himself in charge of over 300 agents and a budget of more than a million dollars and saw in this an opportunity to put his career back on track. Noting a growing agitation in southern states of America about cannabis drugs, he set about gathering negative evidence on the use of cannabis, largely from reports in the newspapers. By 1937 he had succeeded in stoking a media outcry against hemp drugs and had forced the

---

[19] P. Matthews, *Cannabis Culture: A Journey through Disputed Territory* (Bloomsbury, London, 1999), 190–6.

[20] The chief exponent of the conspiracy theory is Jack Herer, *The Emperor Wears No Clothes: Hemp and the Marijuana Conspiracy* (Queen of Clubs Publishing, Van Nuys, Calif., 1992), 24–7.

issue into Congress, where legislation designed to combat consumption of cannabis was passed in 1937.[21] Indeed, so effective was Anslinger in his construction of the case against cannabis and in his orchestration of a media campaign surrounding it that the legislation was passed despite the opposition of the legislative council for the American Medical Association[22] and despite a lack of scientific data and a reliance on uncorroborated newspaper reports.[23]

Historians argue that Anslinger's personal activities would have had little effect had it not been for the culture of the United States in the period. A suspicion of intoxication was a feature of certain American communities in the early twentieth century and indeed this had developed into a dominant theme in the 'Progressive Era' and into the 1920s when agitation for post-First World War moral reform culminated in the prohibition of alcohol.[24] Cannabis itself became closely identified with populations feared by the white legislators of 1930s America as use of the drug was largely associated with Mexican immigrants and Afro-American communities. As such, placing restrictions on the drug was seen as a way of controlling those suspect populations.[25] It was these anxieties about intoxication and about non-white communities that ensured that American newspapers and legislators listened sympathetically to Anslinger's arguments.

Indeed, the politics of the period may also be part of the history of America's legislation on cannabis. The 1930s was the period of the New Deal Congress government in the United States, an administration that was convinced that vigorous state action was the means of solving anything identified as a national evil. As such, it was a government that was receptive to Anslinger's appeal for legislation and for centralized control as it readily agreed that regulations and enforcement were the means of dealing with the problem.[26] Taken together then, the history of the USA's first legislation aimed at curbing the use of cannabis preparations is one of the activities of an entrepreneurial bureaucrat against the backdrop of white America's racist and moralistic attitudes in the context of a control-happy

---

[21] L. Sloman, *The History of Marijuana in America* (Bobbs Merrill, New York, 1979), 31–83.

[22] L. Grinspoon, *Marihuana: The Forbidden Medicine* (Yale University Press, London, 1993), 10–11; A. Mack and J. Joy, *Marijuana as Medicine?* (National Academy Press, Washington, 2001), 158.

[23] For a review of Anslinger's evidence see R. Bonnie and C. Whitebread, *The Marihuana Conviction: A History of Marihuana Prohibition in the United States* (Virginia University Press, Charlottesville, 1974), 154–74.

[24] W. Walker, *Drugs in the Western Hemisphere* (Scholarly Resources, Wilmington, 1996), p. xvi.

[25] Bonnie and Whitebread, *Marihuana Conviction*, 152–3; see also K. Grivas, *Cannabis, Marihuana, Hashish*, trans. D. Whitehouse (Minerva Press, London, 1970), 45–58.

[26] Bonnie and Whitebread, *Marihuana Conviction*, 154.

government. The legislation had no grounds in science or medicine and indeed it has been argued had no grounds in real issues of social order or of crime and punishment.[27]

While the literature available is of little use in providing a detailed history of British policies and laws of the type available on the American position, the media coverage of cannabis offers no more. The *New Scientist* dedicated a whole edition to the subject in 1998 and yet failed to wonder why it was that the policies it produced so much evidence against existed in the first place.[28] A recent study of narcotics in *The Economist* included a short section on the history of drug control that focused largely on America and on opium.[29] The broadsheets and the investigative press have also failed to look in detail at the history of the laws and policies that they are often quick to attack. Instead, these content themselves with accounts that are both inaccurate and fatuous. For example, Howard Marks, the celebrity drug-dealer, was given space in the *Guardian* to write that 'Britannia ruled the waves when dope was last legal. To accommodate the desires of the tobacco, alcohol, pharmaceutical and synthetic fibre industries, an extremely dangerous experiment called cannabis prohibition was imposed on the public during the thirties.'[30] These references to the old conspiracy theories have sometimes been repeated in even greater detail in other news-papers, liberally spiced with other irrelevant nonsense.

Prohibition began in the 1920s thanks to William Randolph Hearst, who wished to use the many acres of forests that he owned to produce paper from wood pulp. He had stitched up a deal with DuPont, who had patented a process to do so, and the only thing left to do was to put marijuana (a new word invented for the purposes of demonizing cannabis) growers out of business—hence the Marijuana Tax. Cotton growers were also happy to jump on the bandwagon.

It could be argued that hemp was responsible for putting the 'Great' into Britain. All rope, sails, and paper required to sustain the British Empire were made from hemp. During the reigns of Henry VIII and Elizabeth I it was possible to be busted for not producing one's tithe of hemp for the realm. What a turn around.[31]

[27] Ibid. 174.
[28] *New Scientist*, 157, 21 Feb. 1998.
[29] 'A Survey of Illegal Drugs', *The Economist*, 28 July 2001.
[30] *Guardian*, 23 Aug. 1997.
[31] Letter in the *Independent*, 18 Oct. 1997.

While the newspapers usually printed incomplete and disjointed versions of the tales told in the books, they did sometimes identify some relevant material:

Western medicine did not discover its benefits until the 1840s. Queen Victoria's physician was one of many who began prescribing it for various illnesses. The growth of jazz clubs in the 1950s and immigration from the West Indies led to its popularity as a recreational drug in this country. Cannabis was outlawed after an Egyptian delegate at an international opium conference in the 1920s made an impassioned plea for Britain to include it in any agreement on the prohibition of opiates. In 1973 the Misuse of Drugs Act outlawed the use of cannabis medicinally. Under the Act it is an offence to allow any premises under your control to be used for growing, preparing, supplying or smoking cannabis.[32]

The problem with such brief accounts is that highlighted above in the case of some of the histories produced by pressure groups and official bodies. These lists may well put their finger on some of the salient facts and information, but while they simply line up the details without any analysis, they leave more questions in the air than they answer.

Despite the ongoing interest in cannabis policies and laws, in government, in the media, by publishers, and among a range of official bodies and pressure groups, there is no detailed account of the origins of those policies and laws and no complete analysis of how those policies and laws came about. This book will therefore tell for the first time the story of the ways in which British governments first formulated procedure and legislation on the issue of cannabis medicines and drugs, and, perhaps more importantly, it will begin to show why they made the decisions they did. Because politicians and policy-makers continue to use history to defend current positions this promises to be a story that reveals much about why Britain has the laws and policies on cannabis that it does today.

[32] 'Potted History', *Independent on Sunday*, 26 Dec. 1999.

2

'Dr O'Shaughnessy appears to have made some experiments with charas': Imperial Merchants, Victorian Science, and Hemp to 1842

GOVERNMENT, HEMP, AND EMPIRE BEFORE 1842

The cannabis plant was a matter of sometimes pressing concern in British government circles from the sixteenth century onwards and by the eighteenth century it was an issue that exercised administrations both in London and across the empire. But the officials and departments that troubled themselves with hemp were not in the least bit interested in its intoxicating properties as their concern was with its fibres.

The reason for this was that it was in this period that Britain was establishing itself as a maritime and imperial power. Rolt's *Dictionary* of 1756 explained that hemp 'is the foundation of several profitable manufactures; as sail cloth, ticking, sacking, cordage, twine and nets: therefore its culture ought to be encouraged, both in Great Britain and its northern colonies in America'.[1] Postlethwayt's *Dictionary* published ten years later was more dramatic: 'our whole mercantile, as well as royal maritime power, depends on supplying ourselves with cordage'.[2] Almost a hundred years later in 1844 it was declared that 'the quantity of hemp used in Great Britain is enormous. The sails and cordage of a ship of war of the first rate require

---

[1] R. Rolt, *A New Dictionary of Trade and Commerce* (London, 1756).
[2] M. Postlethwayt, *The Universal Dictionary of Trade and Commerce* (London, 1766).

180,000 lbs of rough hemp for their construction and it is computed that it takes five acres of land to produce one ton of hemp.'[3] In other words, hemp made up the ropes, rigging, and sails that enabled the ships of the British export/import trade to put to sea in the first place and it could be wound into the bags and the sacks that the country's merchants filled with their booty. Hemp was fundamental to the expanding empire and was central to its technologies.

It is for this reason that Queen Elizabeth I decreed as early as 1563 that landowners with 60 acres or more must grow the hemp plant or face a £5 fine. Such measures proved to be inadequate as by the eighteenth century there was panic in the government on the issue. Lord Somerville, in a letter reproduced in an East India Company report, summarized the importance of finding sources of hemp cordage for the British fleets: 'such are the political relations of Great Britain and such is the unjust as well as unnatural alliance of the Continental Powers against our country that it becomes an imperious duty to make every possible effort to ensure to her that proud security which her maritime force has hitherto commanded and on this account I beg leave to call the most serious attention of the cultivators of our soil to the growth of Hemp'.[4] It was not just the cultivators of Britain whose attention was called to the issue. Reports from Canada and Ireland[5] as well as from India show that the empire was for a time seen as the possible solution to the problem of self-sufficiency in cordage.

Of these reports from the empire the most interesting are those from India that indicate that the British were entirely aware of the local use of hemp for narcotic purposes and that they were increasingly frustrated by this. Robert Wissett, clerk to the Committee of Warehouses of the East India Company, compiled papers on hemp in 1804 which were reprinted in 1808. This research was meant for the Court of Directors of the Company back in London. It seems from this compilation that the Directors had specifically requested this information as the King's Privy Council for Trade and Foreign Plantations had contacted them to request that they consider encouraging the cultivation of hemp in India. Wissett's volume revealed that East India Company representatives in India had already been looking into the question of fibres growing there that might be suitable for cordage. The

[3] *The Dictionary of Trade, Commerce and Navigation* (London, 1844).

[4] 'A Letter from the Rt Hon Lord Somerville on the importance of growing hemp together with an estimate of the expenses', in R. Wissett, *A Treatise on Hemp* (Harding, London, 1808).

[5] P. Besnard, *Observations on Promoting the Cultivation of Hemp and Flax and Extending the Linen and Hempen Manufactures in the South of Ireland* (Folds, Dublin, 1816); C. Taylor, *Remarks on the Culture and Preparation of Hemp in Canada* (Quebec, 1806).

conclusion that they had reached as early as 1801 was that 'the Hemp plant has been cultivated in Bengal from time immemorial for the purpose of intoxication; but is never used by the natives for cordage or cloth as in Europe. The plant is called by them *ganja* and the intoxicating preparation made from it *Bang* [bhang]'.[6] Wissett himself made similar conclusions from his own observations as he noted that

Hemp is not altogether unknown in India but its properties are not sufficiently understood. It is at present cultivated for the purpose of obtaining an intoxicating drug. The substance of which the Natives make their cordage, fishing nets etc. is obtained from a plant called by the Country name SUNN (the crotolaria juncea of Linnaeus) and is prepared in a manner different from the Hemp in Europe. With the view of ascertaining whether this article was capable of being brought into use as a substitute for Hemp, the Board of Trade at Bengal were desirous that a quantity of it should be procured, prepared after the European method; but the Natives were not inclined to depart from their established usage.[7]

The frustration of the British in India came because they failed to persuade Indian producers of hemp to change their cultivation methods to produce a plant that made suitable fibres. An extract from the *Transactions of the Agricultural and Horticultural Society of India*, written over thirty years after Wissett's collection was published, lamented that 'it is well known that no plant is so commonly cultivated in many parts of India as the true Hemp plant which is there called ganja but which differs in no respect from the European plant, though the natives employ it only for the purpose of yielding bhang'.[8] It explained that hemp grown for this purpose was useless for the navy as 'instead of being sown thick as it ought to be when intended for cordages, it is sown thin by the natives who afterwards transplant the young plants and place them at distances of 9 or 10 feet from each other. The effect of this is to expose them more freely to light, heat and air, by the agency of which the plant is enabled to perfect its secretions in a more complete manner and the bhang will consequently be of a more intoxicating nature.' Cultivators in India were uninterested in the cordage crisis of the British Empire as their produce was destined for the cannabis markets of Asia.

The fact that there was such a large trade in cannabis drugs in Asia, and in India in particular, meant that they merited entries in the more specialized publications available for East India Company officers working in the

[6] R. Wissett, *On the Cultivation and Preparation of Hemp* (Cox & Son, London, 1804), 18.
[7] Ibid., p. v.
[8] *Papers Regarding the Cultivation of Hemp in India* (Agra Secundra Orphan Press, 1855), p. iii.

region. These books were important as Company officers were allowed to conduct trade on their own behalf alongside their official duties while they were in Asia. A whole series of regulations evolved to control this personal trade and manuals were published that contained these rules as well as the customs levies payable on personal hoards. Together with these lists of levies and regulations publishers included useful guides to the goods that might be purchased. These guides were intended to help the East India officers work out what was and what was not likely to sell back in Europe and to give them an idea of how to go about buying unfamiliar products without being cheated and without ending up with poor quality samples.

Volumes of this kind provide a fascinating glimpse of the wide variety of articles available to tempt the British trader in his quest to satisfy the European taste for Asian goods. Popular spices included cardamon seeds, 'those produced on the Coast of Malabar are the best',[9] turmeric—'the Bengal sort is not yellow on the outside as the China sort is, but when broke is almost of as good a colour, but very often breaks black'[10]—and cinnamon—'as the Dutch have monopolized this Article...it is hazardous for anyone to buy of them in India the real genuine sorts'.[11] Walking canes from Asia seem to have been popular in Britain by the second half of the eighteenth century as officers were advised to buy them but only if 'sound and heavy, not light and kicksey'.[12] They were a good bet as the King's Duty on them was barely a halfpenny per cane whereas Persian carpets were liable to a levy of over £1 a yard 'which makes them so dear that they are seldom bought'.[13] The more adventurous merchant could buy Dragon's Blood, 'a red resinous gum, sometimes brought in oval lumps, about the size of a chesnut [*sic*] or a Pullet's Egg',[14] hurse skins, 'the Skin of a Fish...chiefly used in Europe to cover small Pocket Cases',[15] or elephants' teeth—'the best should weigh 50lb each'.[16]

Among the range of goods to trade in were the intoxicants of Asia. Opium was defined as 'the concrete juice of the Poppy; it chiefly comes from Turkey, where they prepare it much better than what comes from India, which is much softer and fouler than the Turkey which sometimes come dry enough to break like Spanish Liquorish'.[17] Listed under the

---

[9] H. Adams, *A Short History of Drugs etc. likewise Chinese and Lacquered ware, the produce of the East Indies, published for the sole direction of the commanders and officers in that Service who are allowed private trade, homeward bound* (London, 1779), 15.

[10] Ibid. 34.   [11] Ibid. 54.   [12] Ibid. 57.   [13] Ibid. 60.

[14] Ibid. 17.   [15] Ibid. 62.   [16] Ibid. 61.   [17] Ibid. 47.

heading 'Drugs not much in Demand', opium, the narcotic that was to become so popular in Britain and so important in the economics of the British Empire, was of less interest to the traders of the 1770s than the popular drink arrack. This beverage, 'a fine cane spirit, supposed to be distilled from rice', was described as 'formerly of great Esteem in England but the high duties has lessened the demand, so that fifty or sixty Leagers are sufficient for a Year's consumption'. Traders were warned before speculating as arrack importers that 'what you intend for sale must be full proof, clean, and have no bad smell'.[18]

In 1779 the *Portable Instructions for Purchasing the Drugs and Spices of Asia and the East Indies* gave a rare description of the preparation of cannabis, 'Bangue':

A species of opiate in much repute throughout the East for drowning care. It is the leaf of a kind of wild hemp little differing as to leaf or seed (except in size) from our Hemp. The effects of this drug are to confound the understanding, set the imagination loose and induce a kind of folly or forgetfulness. Mr Grose speaks of it in the following manner: 'Bangue is an intoxicating herb; in the use of which it is hard to say what pleasure can be found, it being very disagreeable to the taste and violent in its operation which produces a temporary madness, that in some, when designedly taken for that purpose, ends in running, what they call a muck, furiously killing every one they meet without distinction till themselves are knocked on the head like mad dogs. But this practice is much rarer in India than it was formerly.[19]

This account of a narcotic preparation of cannabis would have been read by merchants and colonial officers serving in India for well over a century after its publication in 1779. This is because the *Portable Instructions* were regarded as such a useful publication that they were constantly reprinted as an appendix to other guides that were being marketed to those working in Asia. For example, Joseph James and Daniel Moore published *A System of Exchange with almost all Parts of the World* in 1800 and included the *Portable Instructions* under the covers with the title 'The India Directory'.[20] This was a handy pocket-sized book which was designed to provide a means of converting all of the major currencies of international trade into one another. Joseph Huddart's, *The Oriental Navigator or New Direc-*

[18] Ibid. 52.

[19] *Portable Instructions for Purchasing the Drugs and Spices of Asia and the East Indies* (London, 1779), 14.

[20] J. James and D. Moore, *A System of Exchange with almost all Parts of the World. To which is added the India Directory* (John Furman, New York, 1800).

tions for Sailing to and from the East Indies[21] was published in 1801 and also included the *Portable Instructions* appended under the title *The India Officers and Traders Guide in Purchasing the Drugs and Spices of Asia and the East Indies*.

This latter compilation would have guaranteed exposure for the *Portable Instructions* as Huddart's account was the definitive guide to sailing from Britain, France, or America to India. Born in 1740, Captain Joseph Huddart had served with the East India Company since his first voyage as fourth officer on the York in 1773. Despite his father's intention to educate him for the Church, Huddart was at sea by the time he was 20 in the family business of shipping and shipbuilding. He travelled to Ireland, to the Americas, and eventually to Asia, making his fortune as a trader. He filled his time on these voyages as a surveyor and produced the first charts of Sumatra, which were so acclaimed that he was commissioned to produce the most up-to-date survey of the time of the English Channel. His other feats included establishing the most accurate longitude of Bombay for the period, completing surveys of the west coast of India and of the coast of Canton, and organizing the beacons for shipping at Land's End. Such was his celebrity that when the building of the East India docks in London was begun it was he who laid the foundation stone. Huddart's charts and instructions for sailing to, from, and around Asia were the indispensable guides of the period.

Indeed, the continuing popularity of the volume containing Huddart's guides bound together with *The India Officers and Traders Guide in Purchasing the Drugs and Spices of Asia and the East Indies* is demonstrated by its constant use. The copy in the British Library shows that it had at least three owners during its working life. E. N. Skerry wrote his name in the cover on November 1824 and another Skerry, no doubt a relative of the first signatory, signed himself S. W. Skerry in 1860. A final owner, a Harold E. Gibbs, decided that the book was important enough a possession to stamp his ownership on in 1917 as it was signed in that year in his neat and rather fancy handwriting. The *Portable Instructions*, first published in 1779 and bound up with Huddart's charts as *The India Officers and Traders Guide* in 1801, were still in use almost a century and a half later during the First World War.

If at any point in that century or so the owners of the book decided to consult it for information on cannabis preparations then they would have

---

[21] J. Huddart, *The Oriental Navigator or New Directions for Sailing to and from the East Indies* was published in the United States in 1801 with *The India Officers and Traders Guide in Purchasing the Drugs and Spices of Asia and the East Indies* (James Humphreys, Philadelphia, 1801).

found that the entry was heavily reliant on the opinions of 'Mr Grose'. This authority was in fact John-Henry Grose, the author of *A Voyage to the East Indies with Observations on Various Parts there* published in 1757.[22] He sailed in 1750 as a writer in the East India Company, the equivalent of an administrative manager in the firm. His book was to become popular enough to go into an expanded edition in 1766 and a third edition in 1772 as well as to be translated into French in 1758.

Much of the apparent popularity of the book can be explained by its parochial Englishness, as the tone throughout is one that would have confirmed the reader in a sense of the decadently exotic nature of India and the superior state of the English. The Mahrattas were a 'civilized nation of banditti', the Mughal Emperor 'no more than a phantom on the throne', and the Brahmins and Banyans, the priests and moneylenders of India, 'do not want for that vice of cowards, vindictiveness'. Stories of sex, superstition, and intoxication filled the pages. For example, Grose seemed much taken with the dancing-girls of the Mughal court:

They, as well as other women in that country, have a peculiar way of managing and preserving their breasts which at the same time makes no inconsiderable part of their finery. They enclose them in a pair of hollow cups or cases exactly fitted to them, made of a very light wood, linked together, and buckle at the back. These at once confine the breasts so as that they cannot grow to any disgustfully exuberant size, and yet, from their smoothness and pliancy, play so freely with every motion of the body, that they do not crush the exquisitely tender texture of the flesh in that part.

Drunkenness was part of the portrait that Grose painted of high society in India and he delighted in the unfamiliar methods of distilling in the region. He described the 'various strong spirits, to which they give names that would seem odd, such as spirit of mutton, spirit of deer, spirit of goat, but for the reason they annex to it, which is their throwing into the still according to the liquor they propose, a joint of mutton, a haunch of venison, a quarter of a goat, which give respectively their names to the distillation. This they imagine, how justly I do not pretend to know, super-adds to the liquor a certain mellowness and softness, that corrects the fieriness of the spirit.' It seems that Mr Grose was a little more reluctant to try the local drinks than he was to sample the local dancing-girls.

Drugs were another part of the picture that Grose created of the licentious Indian rulers. Opium was a favourite, and of course in Grose's

[22] J. Grose, *A Voyage to the East Indies with Observations on Various Parts there* (Hooper & Morley, London, 1757).

account it had to have sexual links. He assured the reader that 'many of the rich and great too contract a habit of it, considering it not only as a high point of sensuality, from the pleasing deliriums they experience from it, but as a specific for procuring a priapism that serves to spin out the venereal congress as long as they please'. Then of course there were his opinions of the cannabis preparation 'Bang'. He asserted that 'Bang is also greatly used at Surat, as well as all over the East' before going on to make his claims, quoted in full above from the *Portable Instructions*, that 'it is hard to say what pleasure can be found in the use of it, being very disagreeable to the taste, and violent in its operation'.

It is difficult however to claim that Grose's account of cannabis, or indeed of India, is reliable or accurate and much easier to conclude that it was never his intention to produce information that was any of these things. The book seems to be written in order to appeal to his audience and the List of Subscribers that bought the first edition suggests that this was a fairly representative slice of eighteenth-century, middle-class England. The Reverend Mr Fermer Maltus of Shooter Hill took a copy, as did Mrs Gaudy, mistress of the Boarding School at Richmond, and Mr Richard Capell, a surgeon at Bermondsey. Mr John Watson, surgeon on the Royal Carolina, no doubt enjoyed passing his time at sea with the spicy reading provided by Mr Grose, and Lieutenant William Meldrum was sufficiently excited to order two copies in advance. Such an audience's predilection for titillating tales of oriental excess and for reassuring paragraphs on 'the mildness and tolerance of the English government' suggests that John Henry Grose would have carefully selected and embellished his stories rather than simply presented a balanced view of all that he witnessed in Asia. Grose made an association between cannabis drugs, violence, madness, and death which had these questionable origins. Nevertheless, this association remained the basis of the information available to British officers and other merchants on cannabis in the *Portable Instructions* that continued to be used into the twentieth century.

On the whole then, the evidence suggests that before the middle of the nineteenth century hemp products figured in the concerns of British government largely because of the problems of securing cordage for the country's navies and commercial activities. Officials both in the UK and in the colonies wrote lengthy reports on the subject and the empire was for a time considered a potential solution to the demand for strong and flexible materials until it became obvious in the early nineteenth century that hemp was a source of drugs rather than fibres in India. In the books written by and for merchants and traders there is only a vague awareness of the intoxicating properties of hemp, such as the note in Rolt's *Dictionary of Trade and Commerce* of 1756 that mentioned that 'its leaves arise by fives, or sixes from the same pedicle, and are a little jagged; yielding a strong smell which affects the head'.[23] The most colourful accounts of the drug, which were included in some of the most popular travelling companion guides of the period, were given by John-Henry Grose, who hoped to amuse his audience rather than to accurately inform them. What all the accounts of hemp do show however is that of all the places in the world that British administrators and merchants were trading in and travelling to, it was in India that their awareness of hemp narcotics was being formed.

MEDICAL MEN, SCIENTIFIC KNOWLEDGE, AND CANNABIS DRUGS BEFORE 1842

It was the medical men and scientists of the East India Company that devoted most interest to cannabis drugs before the middle of the nineteenth century. Medical publications from the 1700s show that there was an awareness of the properties of the hemp plant that meant that it could be used both as a medicine and as an intoxicant. However, the nature of the entries in these books points to the fact that there was little direct experience of the medicinal preparations of the plant. Pocket guidebooks available for the layman such as John Jacob Berlu's *The Treasury of Drugs Unlocked* relayed the information that 'Bang' was 'an herb which comes from Bantam in the East Indies of an infatuating quality and pernicious use'.[24] Berlu, a London drugs merchant, obviously did not approve of hemp products but it is doubtful that he had encountered them much as he listed 'Bang' as one of the substances prohibited by the government. These substances were prohibited not because of their perceived effects but because of the Navigation Acts.

These Acts had been introduced in the reign of Charles II to regulate the trade of the King's territories. The Acts, in the words of Parliament, aimed to ensure that 'no goods or commodities whatsoever shall be imported into or exported out of any lands, islands, plantations or territories to his majesty belonging, or in his possession, or which may hereafter belong unto or be in the possession of his Majesty, his heirs and successors in Asia, Africa, or

---

[23] Rolt, *A New Dictionary of Trade and Commerce.*
[24] J. Berlu, *The Treasury of Drugs Unlocked or a Full and True Description of Drugs, Chymical Preparations Sold by Druggists* (Ballard, London, 1738).

America in any other ship or ships, vessel or vessels whatsoever, but in such ships or vessels as do truly, and without fraud, belong only to the people of England, or Ireland, dominion of Wales or Town of Berwick upon Tweed, or are of the built of, and belonging to and the said lands, islands, plantations or territories'.[25] Quite simply, these Acts sought to guarantee that all trade in and out of England and its empire after 1660 was carried in ships that were owned by the King's subjects.

Berlu noted that bhang was associated with Bantam. Bantam, now part of Indonesia, was at that time under the influence of the Dutch rather than the British East India Company as the former had sided with the victorious rebels in the civil war in Bantam of the 1680s. As such, by 1684[26] the exports of the region would have been carried to Europe in Dutch rather than British shipping. Under the Navigation Acts this would have meant that they would have been illegal in Britain as goods 'being not brought directly from the place of growth in English built shipping'[27] were prohibited. Cannabis seems to have been illegal in the UK as early as the 1680s then, not because of its effects, but because it was the product of a rival Asian empire.

Indeed, an intriguing passage in the Preface to Berlu's handbook suggests that the author himself had fallen foul of the Navigation Acts. In dedicating the book to the 'Courteous and Benevolent Reader' he outlined the objectives of his publication. He hoped to promote trade and to banish ignorance, but he also declared that he was keen for others 'to avoid also those dangers (of prohibited goods) by which I have been (as it were) shipwracked, you will easily discern the places of growth, being mentioned almost to every commodity, and thereby avoid those rocks and perils by which I have forgone a good estate'. It is difficult to trace the history of the case of John Jacob Berlu but he seems to be complaining that for want of the sort of guide that he had written he had fallen foul of the Navigation Acts by buying products that were prohibited. This handy guide, first published in 1690 but reprinted in 1738, seems to have been written by a victim of some of Britain's earliest drug laws.

The more specialist medical publications of the eighteenth century do carry greater detail but again reveal that in the period there was little direct British experience of hemp substances. The massive three volumes of *A*

[25] *A Subsidy granted to the king of tonnage and poundage and other sums of mony payable upon merchandize exported and imported* (Bill & Barker, London, 1667).
[26] C. Boxer, *The Dutch Seaborne Empire, 1600–1800* (Hutchinson, London, 1977), 198.
[27] Berlu, *The Treasury of Drugs Unlocked.*

Medicinal Dictionary[28] compiled by Robert James and printed by the Society of Booksellers for Promoting Learning were intended to be a compilation of all knowledge relating to 'Physic, Surgery, Anatomy, Chymistry and Botany in all their branches relative to medicine together with a history of drugs, an account of their various preparations, combinations, and uses'. The collection included a dedication written by Samuel Johnson, who of course was to go on to write his own dictionary of the English language, and who wrote some of the entries in the *Medicinal Dictionary*.

The entries on cannabis and on 'bangue' show considerable confusion as to the properties of these substances. 'Bangue' is given a number of interesting Latin names, *cannabis fimilis exotica* or *cannabis indica trifoliate* but it is not identified as a preparation of Hemp (cannabis sativa). Instead it is described as 'almost like Hemp' but it is clearly stated that 'it is a different plant from Hemp'. The *Medicinal Dictionary* notes no medical uses of 'Bangue' and instead focuses on the leisure pursuits in which the preparation featured.

The Indians, says Acosta, eat the seed and leaves to increase their vigour in love affairs and to excite an appetite to their food. The nobles, and chief military officers, when they are disposed to forget their toil and to sleep in perfect ease and security, take of the powder of the seed and leaves as much as they think sufficient and thereto add an Areca or green Indian hazel-nut and as much opium as they think fit and eat them all together with sugar. If they desire to be entertained with variety of scenes and images of things in their sleep they add some of the choicest camphire, cloves, nutmegs and mace. If they have a mind to be merry, witty, and to indulge their amours they add Ambergrise and musk and make them all an electuary with sugar.

On the other hand the entry for cannabis sativa points out that 'it has been formerly believed to render Persons unactive in Venereal Affairs; but that is not at all likely, for it not only causes Hens to lay Eggs in Plenty, if given moderately; but the famous Bangue so much used by Persians and Indians to promote Venery, is a Species of Hemp'. The relationship between bhang and hemp is here identified but it is decided that they are different parts of the same family. The entry under cannabis sativa does note a variety of medicinal uses, 'the juice of the green plant, instil'd into the Ears, mitigates the Pains therein' and 'the seed of the Hemp which is the only part used in Physic, being boiled in Milk till it cracks is accounted good for old coughs, and a specific to cure the Jaundice'.

[28] R. James, *A Medicinal Dictionary* ... (Osborne, London, 1745).

James's dictionary demonstrates that while there was knowledge in the British medical profession in the UK of certain cannabis preparations and the medicinal and narcotic uses to which they were put there was also a large amount of confusion and a distinct lack of precision about this knowledge. This did not stop the James entry on cannabis becoming established as authoritative and the more general encyclopedias that flourished later in the eighteenth century reproduced the details word for word. *The Complete Dictionary of Arts and Sciences* published in 1765 for example began its section on 'Hemp', to which those seeking information on 'Cannabis' were directed, with the sentence 'cannabis, in botany, a very useful plant for making cordage and all things of that kind',[29] which were the exact words at the start of the James entry.

The confusion and lack of precision in these details can be explained by the fact that there was little direct experience of cannabis preparations among British doctors and as such they were reliant on questionable sources of information. Most of the entries on bhang quoted Dioscorides and Acosta as the authorities. Dioscorides was a Greek physician whose list of medicinal herbs and their virtues had remained an authority since it was compiled in the first century AD. Cristoval Acosta was a sixteenth-century Spanish medical man from Burgos who had written a treatise on medicines and drugs in India back in 1578. He had met Garcie d'Orta, who first sailed for Goa from Portugal in 1534 and who was to serve as doctor to the Portuguese Viceroys of India for over thirty years until his death in 1568. D'Orta was a colourful character who, as the son of Jewish converts to Christianity, emigrated to the empire to escape the Inquisition. Once in India, he readily befriended Muslims and Hindus and happily chatted with local shopkeepers and chemists in order to explore the secrets of Asian medicines. He never himself went further from the Portuguese colonies than Ahmadnagar or Sri Lanka but he did organize a network of correspondents further afield to send him samples and seeds of medicinal plants. He died a rich man, one of the first Europeans to own the island that is now Bombay, but he ultimately fell foul of the Inquisition, which ordered some twelve years after his death that his remains be exhumed and burnt as a Christaos-Novos (Jewish convert).[30]

---

[29] T. Croker et al., *The Complete Dictionary of Arts and Sciences in which the Whole Circle of Human Learning is Explained* (London, 1765).

[30] C. Boxer, *Two Pioneers of Tropical Medicine: Garcia d'Orta and Nicolas Monardes* (Wellcome, London, 1963), 7–11.

D'Orta has been credited as the first European to compile an Indian *materia medica* and as early as 1619 was described as 'le premier qui avec loüange a frayé le sentier de la cognoissance des medicaments és Indes Orientales'.[31] His 'Coloquios dos simples e drogas he cousas medicinais da India'[32] are certainly the earliest colonial European writings on South Asian medicine by a western doctor who had direct contact with Indian society. His original papers were in Portuguese but his compilation was seen as important enough to be translated into Latin and later into French.[33] In it there is a lengthy entry on cannabis products.

As many are of the opinion that the bangue of Indians does not differ from opium that they call ofium through a corruption of the word, it does not seem without purpose to say something about Bangue.

Bangue, therefore, is a plant that does not badly resemble hemp, as its seeds are a little smaller and not as white; furthermore its woody shoots are not covered with any husk, which appears totally in contrast to hemp. Finally, the Indians eat the leaves and the seed of the same to render them more inclined to the venereal act; considering which the Authorities attribute to it the opposite power of the seeds of hemp, which have the power to dry out the genital seed.

The juice is expressed from the pounded leaves and sometimes also from the seeds to which some add a very tart baste (because it somewhat intoxicates and hurts the brain's senses) or some nutmeg, some mace, sometimes cloves, as well as some Borneo camphor; others add amber and musc, and much opium, like the richest and most opulent of the Moors. They receive no other benefit than this, they are as if ravished in ecstacy and delivered from all thoughts and cares, and they laugh at the least thing that they see.

Moreover, I can say that I first came across its use for this purpose among the officers of the armies and other soldiers, who wearied through constant vigilance, have drunk some of this bangue with wine, or with opium, and have talked as if drunk, and sleep deeply as if delivered from all cares.

As the great Sultan Badur was accustomed to say to Martin Alphonse de Sousa, the King's Counsellor, whom he liked very much, and to whom he told his most secret plans, when he dreamed of going to Portugal, to Brazil, to Asia Minor, to Arabia, or to Persia, he need only take a little bangue, with some sugar, and he would mingle in the places that he had mentioned; they call this mixture *maju*.

---

[31] A. Colin (ed.), *Histoire des drogues, espiceries et de certains medicamens simples qui naissent es Indes et en l'Amerique* (Pillehotte, Lyon, 1619), 3; 'the first who, praise him, trod the path of knowledge of the medicines of the Oriental Indies'.

[32] G. D'Orta, *Coloquios dos simples e drogas he cousas medicinais da India* (Ioannes Goa, 1563). I am very grateful to Tom Dodd for the excellent translation.

[33] G. du Iardin (French spelling of G. D'Orta), *Histoire de quelques plantes des Indes*, in A. Colin (ed.), *Histoire des drogues*, 3.

Cristoval Acosta claims to have met d'Orta while in India and to have
been inspired by his writings and the outcome was his own volume on the
natural history of India. Again, it seems certain that Acosta was recording his
own personal investigations and experiences of medicines and drugs as he was
keen to emphasize that he was writing about 'what I myself have seen, on long
and various journeys, that which others have put in writing only on hear-say'.
Indeed, he even boasted that his account corrected the writings of the traditional Greek, Latin, and Arab authorities on drugs, which he claimed were
littered with errors that he put down to the authors having relied on second-
hand reports. The work was certainly considered to be significant enough to
be translated from Spanish into Latin within four years of its original publication in 1578, into Italian for the Venetians in 1585 and into French in 1619.
On the subject of 'Bangue', however, his entry, which was to be the source for
the James *Dictionary*, relied heavily on the account of d'Orta.

Bangue almost resembles hemp, which Dioscorides mentioned in his third
volume. Its stalk is of a height of two and a half feet, carries a bright green colour,
is difficult to break, is not as hollowed as the stalk of the hemp, the skin of which
also serves well as a fibre like that of hemp; its leaves are like those of hemp. Green
and tall, and at the base hairy and white, of a weak and earthy taste: its seed is also
smaller than that of hemp and is not as white.

The Indians eat the seed and the leaves in order to render themselves fit for the
venereal act and to encourage the appetite. Of this bangue one makes a mixture
that is largely used in these countries for many maladies; also the nobles and
military officers, to the end of sleeping more securely and freely, and to forget their
troubles, take their dose of the powder of the leaves and the seed and add some
Areca, or green Indian filbeard and some opium according to taste: they eat all of
this with sugar: if they desire to see lots of dreams and illusions while sleeping they
add some of the choicest camphire, cloves, nutmegs and mace: if they want to be
merry, witty, and are inclined to carnal delights, they add Ambergrise and musk
and prepare an electuary.

Many have assured me that the leaves and seeds of this plant, are of a marvellous
effectiveness and prowess for inciting carnal delights (fleshlinesse); on which one
can be assured that it has not any affinity or relation to hemp, to which it has a
strong resemblance, seeing that Dioscorides has instead argued that hemp is hot
and dry and extinguishes genital seed.

The Arabs call it Axis, the Persians, those of the Deccan and many other
regions call it bangue, and the Turks Asarath.[34]

[34] C. Acosta, *Des drogues et medicaments qui naissent aux Indes*, in A. Colin (ed.), *Histoire des drogues*, 157–9. I am very grateful to Tom Dodd for the excellent translation.

It is evident from comparing these accounts with that of James's *Medicinal Dictionary* that eighteenth-century Englishmen liked the stories about soldiers, sex, and sleep told by the sixteenth-century Iberians and enthusiastically reproduced them. The entry on 'bangue' in the James *Dictionary*, however, did also rely on more contemporary sources. For example, the description is careful to mention the opinion of Sir Hans Sloane. Sloane was the major medical figure of the period when James's *Dictionary* was published. He treated Queen Anne and King George II, succeeded Isaac Newton as president of the Royal Society, and founded the British Museum, as well as giving his name to Sloane Street and Sloane Square in London. His interest in natural history was such that he founded the Chelsea Botanical Garden and had a personal library of over 42,000 books that was described as 'the fullest and most curious in the world, with regard to the several branches of natural history and physick'.[35] No doubt his conclusions were included in order to give the most up-to-date impressions of a major medical and botanical English authority. There is no evidence however that Sloane had had any direct experience of cannabis sativa and his assertion that 'bangue' 'is a different plant from Hemp' is of course wrong.

The extract did also credit Philip Miller with the conclusion 'the famous Bangue so much used by Persians and Indians to promote Venery, is a Species of Hemp'. Britain's first celebrity gardener, Philip Miller tended to the beds of Sir Hans Sloane, was a member of the Royal Society, and published *The Gardener's Dictionary* in 1724. Miller's major published work, however, suggests that he was little interested in hemp and was unconcerned with its intoxicating properties. He was credited with writing the botanical entries in the *Dictionarium Britannicum*, one of the earlier eighteenth-century attempts to compile an English language dictionary. Hemp seemed not to have captured his curiosity as the entry simply read 'a sort of coarse flax'.[36] Indeed, the *Gardener's Dictionary* was hardly more illuminating and betrayed little inspiration, although he did at least show an awareness of the plant's variety of uses.

This Plant is propogated in the rich fenny parts of Lincolnshire in great quantities for its bark which is so useful for cordage, cloth etc and the seeds afford an oyl

---

[35] *A Concise Narrative of the Life, Travels, Collections, Works etc. of Sir Hans Sloane* (Cooper, London, 1755), 50.

[36] N. Bailey, *Dictionarium Britannicum or a Compleat Universal Etymological English Dictionary* (Cox, London, 1730).

which is used in medecine. The manner of propogating it is so well known that it would be needless to insert it in this place.[37]

Later editions of the *Gardener's Dictionary*, prepared after the death of Philip Miller by Thomas Martyn who was a Professor of Botany at Cambridge, did expand on hemp but again there seemed to be little direct experience of hemp's narcotic properties to flesh out the entry. The 1807 edition devoted most of its attention to the 'manner of propogating it' that Miller had not bothered to detail in his original entries. Indeed the medicinal uses alluded to in the original had disappeared by the nineteenth century as Martyn simply notes 'an oil is extracted from the seeds of hemp' without repeating the words 'which is used in medecine' that Miller had included in his *Dictionary*. In place of the observation of medicinal use there was a fanciful tale repeated without any substantiation about birds: 'the seeds themselves are reckoned a good food for poultry and are supposed to occasion hens to lay a greater quantity of eggs. Small birds in general are very fond of them but they should be given to caged birds with caution and mixed with other feeds. A very singular effect is recorded on very good authority to have been sometimes produced by feeding Bullfinches and Goldfinches on hemp-feed alone or in too great quantity; viz that of changing the red and yellow on those birds to a total blackness.'[38]

In short, there is little evidence of direct experience in British medical and scientific circles of intoxicating cannabis preparations before the nineteenth century. While many of the textbooks of the time prove that there was an awareness of such preparations they seem to rely on second-hand information or the speculation of eighteenth-century experts. The most recent direct contact referred to in those textbooks was that of the Spanish and Portuguese doctors Acosta and d'Orta whose information had come from personal enquiries in India.

It seems that it was India then that was the source of information on hemp drugs for the scientists and doctors of Britain, as it was for the merchants and administrators of the empire. Indeed, information gathered by British scientists on medicinal plants in other parts of the world failed to mention the hemp plant altogether. Hans Sloane, already noted above as one of the key British natural scientists of the eighteenth century, had direct medical knowledge of the Caribbean Islands and had brought with him

[37] P. Miller, *The Gardener's Dictionary, containing the methods of cultivating and improving the kitchen, fruit and flower garden as also the physick garden, wilderness, conservatory and vineyard* (Rivington, London, 1731).

[38] T. Martyn, *The Gardener's and Botanist's Dictionary by the late Philip Miller, The whole corrected and newly arranged* (Rivington et al., London, 1807).

from his travels there a collection of over 800 plant specimens. However, it does not seem that hemp or 'bangue' were included in this as there is no mention of the plant in the voluminous 'Natural History of the Herbs and Trees, four-footed beasts, fishes, birds, insects, reptiles etc.' that was appended to his account of his time abroad.[39] Over a hundred years later a subsequent British study of plant life in Jamaica similarly failed to note cannabis in the local flora.[40]

It was not until the nineteenth century that British scientists and doctors in India began to report their own experiences with these substances. One of the earliest of these reports and perhaps one of the most important of the early nineteenth century was that of Whitelaw Ainslie. He published the following account of 'Ganjah' in 1813.

Ganjah (Tamil, Duk and Malay), Kanub (Arab), Hemp Cannabis Sativa, Vijya, Sanjica (Sanskrit).

Ganjah is the Tamool name of the plant from which Bangie and Majum are prepared.

The leaves are frequently added to tobacco and smoked to increase its intoxicating power; they are also sometimes, given in cases of Diarrhoea and in conjunction with Turmeric, Onions and warm Ginglie oil, are made into an application for painful, swelled and protruded Piles. In Malays this plant is called Ginji Lacki Lucki; it is the Kalengi Cansjava of the Hortus Malabaricus.[41]

Elsewhere he included an entry to cover the substances 'Bangie' and 'Majum' that he had mentioned here: 'Majum: This electuary is much used by the Mahometans particularly the more dissolute who take it internally to intoxicate and ease pain and not unfrequently from an overdose of it, produce a temporary mental derangement. The chief ingredients employed in making it are Gunjah leaves, Milk, Ghee, Poppy Seeds, Flowers of the Thorn Apple, the powder of the Nux Vomica and Sugar. Another inebriating preparation made with the leaves of the Gunjah plant is Bang or Bengie. It is in liquid form and is chiefly drank by the Mahometans and Mahrattas; the Tamools and Telingas who are comparatively temperate and circumspect, use it but little.'[42]

---

[39] H. Sloane, *A Voyage to the Islands of Madera, Barbados, Nieves, S. Christophers and Jamaica* (London, 1707).

[40] John Lunan, *Hortus Jamaicensis or a botanical description (according to the Linnean system) and an account of the virtues etc of its indigenous plants hitherto known as also of the most useful exotics compiled from the best authorities and alphabetically arranged in two volumes* (St Jago de la Vega Gazette, 1814).

[41] W. Ainslie, *Materia Medica of Hindoostan and Artisan's and Agriculturist's Nomenclature* (Government Press, Madras, 1813), 80.

[42] Ibid. 86.

The significance of these entries was that they came in the 'Materia Medica of Hindoostan' that Ainslie had prepared while he was a Superintending Surgeon in Madras. This was the first attempt by a British colonial official to take on the task, attempted back in the sixteenth century by the Spanish and Portuguese doctors da Costa and d'Orta, of compiling a list of drugs and medicines used in India. He had worked in close conjunction with a British botanist in India, the Reverend Doctor J. P. Rottler, who granted access to the garden at St Thomas's Mount in Madras. The importance of the project is underlined by the fact that the Government Press took on the job of publishing the volume by special permission of the government itself.

The entry on ganja was careful to point out that Indians did use preparations of the cannabis plant for specifically medical reasons, for piles and diarrhoea and more generally to ease pain. However, the balance of the reports was towards the use of hemp substances for their 'intoxicating power'. Little had changed thirteen years later when Ainslie published a revised and expanded two-volume series, this time with the title *Materia Indica*.[43] The information on bhang and majum was much the same, although each had been given a separate entry in the collection. The entry on 'ganja' was noticeably longer than in the original edition. Much of it was dedicated to a debate about the origin of the plant and Ainslie summarized the opinions of those that were sure that it came from Persia, Europe, 'Tartary', or even Japan. Significantly, however he expanded the account of the use by Indians of preparations of ganja for intoxicating purposes, 'though some people have bestowed on the plant now under our notice the botanical appellation of cannabis Indica; yet as it does not appear except in size to differ at all from the cannabis sativa of Europe, we have retained the original specific name. It would seem however to be applied to very different purposes in Eastern countries from those for which it is resorted to in colder territories; being chiefly employed in the former for its inebriating and narcotic qualities.' His account of the love of Indians for intoxication through the drug was backed up by quoting the conclusions of others:

I understand that in some districts of central India cordage and a coarse kind of cloth are occasionally prepared with it; in Nepaul too, by Kirkpatrick's account of that country, it would seem that linens and sackcloth are sometimes made with it;

[43] W. Ainslie, *Materia Indica or some account of those articles which are employed by the Hindoos and other eastern nations in their medicine, arts and agriculture* (Longman, Rees, Orme, Brown & Green, London, 1826).

the Chinese from what Barrow says use it little for such purposes but are acquainted with its intoxicating powers. The Malays, Crawfurd informs us, cultivate the plant only for smoking. The Turks know well its stupefying effects and
call it Malach. Linnaeus speaks of its 'vis narcotica, phantastica, dementens,
anodyna et repellens'. It would appear that even the Hottentots use it to get drunk
with and call it dacha. We are told by Avicenna that the seeds of the cannabis
sativa are termed by the Arabians [*sic*] and that the inebriating substance prepared
from the bruised leaves they name hushish.

Indeed, Ainslie was eager to add to the air of strange and exotic properties that he attached to cannabis by observing that 'Miller notices some
curious, perhaps absurd circumstances respecting the seed; such as that
when eaten by fowls they make them lay many eggs; and that when
bullfinches and goldfinches take them in considerable quantity as food,
they have the effect of changing the red and yellow of those birds to total
blackness. No oil is extracted from them in India.' This extract showed
that he had turned to the revised 1807 version of Philip Miller's *Gardener's
Dictionary* for information as this tale had first appeared there. Despite all
this, Ainslie did also expand his observations on the medicinal uses of
ganja. Significantly, this was by way of only a short sentence that appeared
at the end of those lengthy passages exploring the intoxicating and mysterious character of hemp substances. 'Some of the Hakeems of the lower
provinces are in the habit of preparing with the seeds a kind of emulsion
which they prescribe in gonorrhoea' was all that he was prepared to admit.

Ainslie's revised account very much lay the emphasis on the use of ganja
as a means of intoxication rather than as a useful medicine. This decision to
focus on the non-medicinal uses of cannabis preparations may well be
explained by the author's interests outside medical science. He was, of
course, a significant medical scientist in the early nineteenth century and
indeed he was knighted for his services in this capacity and received com-
mendations from the East India Company for his work on cholera. He
was, however, also a committed Christian who moved in a circle of mis-
sionaries and who was the author of a range of publications with moral and
religious content.

A good example of these would be his *An Historical Sketch of the Introduction of Christianity into India and its Progress and Present State in that and other
Eastern Countries*, which was published by Oliver & Boyd in Edinburgh in
1835. The objective of this book was to examine strands of Christianity in
India, a country for which Ainslie evidently had much affection, having
served there for almost thirty years. But in the book he betrayed a distinctly
unscientific nature, lauding the 'sacred truths first brought into the world

by our Redeemer; that merciful being who, by MIRACULOUSLY[44] healing the corporeal infirmities of men, gave promise of that yet more exalted power, by which he could heal the souls as well as bodies of such as might faithfully believe in him'.[45] His commitment was to what he called in another of his publications 'the bless'd reward of *Persevering Virtue*'[46] that grew from his Christian beliefs. An ability to resist the temptations of wordly pleasures was part and parcel of the nineteenth-century Christian zealot's commitment to 'persevering virtue' and it is evident that Ainslie certainly approved of this, as he asked in defending India from its critics 'where is there such habitual temperance? In England? No!'[47]

Indeed, his chapter in the *Historical and Descriptive Account of British India* emphasizes his commitment to a frugal and disciplined lifestyle that points to little patience for those that chose to indulge freely in pleasures of the body. This three-volume collection in the Edinburgh Cabinet Library series of publications was designed to be a comprehensive introduction to India and the third volume contained essays on such topics as disease, climate, and geography. Sir Whitelaw Ainslie contributed the entry on 'Constitutions best suited to India, preservation of health on board ship and after arrival, management after return to Europe'. In this he made clear that

This is no place to treat medically of indigestion; yet it may not be amiss to warn all young Eastern adventurers who wish to avoid it that they will do wisely to live on the plainest food, which should be well done; to dine, if possible, on one dish, or two dishes at most; not to take more than two meals in the day, the second certainly not sooner than six hours after the first; not to be afraid of black tea, which, in moderation is virtually stomachic; to masticate sufficiently so as not to entail on the stomach a duty which does not belong to it; to shun crude vegetables or fruits; to prefer that liquor (sparingly used) which is least apt to produce acidity, such as Cape Madeira of the best quality, sherry or weak brandy and water; not to expose themselves to great heat more than duty requies; to sleep with the head high; to take care that the bowels are kept regularly open; and if their situation renders it convenient to use equitation (of all the modes of exercise the most conducive to health in India is riding on horseback) in the cool of the morning.

[44] Emphasis in original.

[45] W. Ainslie, *An Historical Sketch of the Introduction of Christianity into India and its Progress and Present State in that and other Eastern Countries* (Oliver & Boyd, Edinburgh, 1835), 15–16.

[46] W. Ainslie, *Clemenza or The Tuscan Orphan: A Tragic Drama in Five Acts* (Cruttwell, Bath, 1822), 93.

[47] Ainslie, *Historical Sketch*, 143.

A simple and temperate lifestyle was recommended by the man who had served thirty years in India and who lived to be 69. When his entry on cannabis preparations is looked at again in the knowledge that he was writing as a committed Victorian Christian who considered frugality to be the path to 'perservering virtue' it seems unsurprising, but also rather unscientific, that he included information that seemed to neglect the medicinal properties of the plant and instead focused on the intoxication and intemperance that he so disapproved of.

Indeed, other publications on the subject by British scientists of the nineteenth century seem to be open to the same criticism, that they were written by men whose religious and moral commitments meant that they saw the plant's intoxicating properties as a potential source of sin. The Edinburgh Cabinet Library *Historical and Descriptive Account of British India* also had a chapter titled 'An Account of a few of the more remarkable Indian plants in which the species are arranged according to the natural families to which they belong'. The author of this essay was Dr Robert Kaye Greville, one of the great botanists of the nineteenth century who had published in 1831 a collection of over 200 drawings of Indian plants (based on samples sent to him by Nathaniel Wallich in India rather than on personal travel) and who was to go on to serve as an MP for Edinburgh in 1856. Under the *Urtica* family section he included a lengthy entry on cannabis sativa. He was adamant that 'cannabis sativa, or the common hemp, another plant of this family, is less well known out of Europe for its useful fibre than the intoxicating and stupifying qualities of its leaves'.[48] His account however, went on to rely on other sources but he was sure that 'it was formerly put to the vilest of purposes'. This was the same Robert Kaye Greville that was the editor of a Scottish version of the Church of England hymn book in 1838 and who dashed off pamphlets such as 'Facts Illustrative of the Drunkenness of Scotland with observations on the responsibility of the clergy, magistrates, and other influential bodies of the community' to remind all of their responsibilities to control intemperance and intoxication. Indeed, his obituary insisted that 'when the temperance reform was first introduced into the country he gave up a large portion of time to it for several years and addressed innumerable meetings on the subject'.[49] There is therefore good reason to doubt the extent to which the author was likely to

[48] R. Greville, 'Some account of a few of the more remarkable Indian plants in which the species are arranged according to the natural families to which they belong', in H. Murray et al. (eds.), *Historical and Descriptive Account of British India* (Oliver & Boyd, Edinburgh, 1832).
[49] J. Balfour, 'Obituary Notice of Dr Greville', in *The Collected Works of Dr RK Greville on Diatomaceae* (Neill, Edinburgh, 1866), 13.

produce a balanced account of a substance that produced the inebriation to which he was so personally opposed.

Greville had taken much of his information from John Forbes Royle's *Illustrations of the Botany and other Branches of the Natural History of the Himalayan Mountains and of the Flora of Cashmere*,[50] which was published in 1839 and which was the result of the author's personal observations while stationed at Saharunpore, where he was the superintendent of the East India Company's botanical garden. However, Greville had been selective in lifting information from this volume as while Royle was aware that the plant was often used in making intoxicating substances he was keen to point to its other uses in India and certainly had not written as had Greville that hemp 'is less well known out of Europe for its useful fibre than the intoxicating and stupifying qualities of its leaves'. Royle had indeed composed the passage that Greville quoted and which detailed the intoxicating substances derived from hemp.

A peculiar substance is yielded by the plants in the hills, in the form of a glandular secretion, which is collected by the natives pressing the upper part of the growing plant between the palms of their hands, and then scraping off the secretion which adheres. This is well known in India by the name cherris and is considered more intoxicating than any other preparation of this plant, which is so highly esteemed by many Asiatics, serving them both for wine and opium; it has in consequence a variety of names applied to it in Arabic, some of which were translated to me as 'grass of fuqueers', 'leaf of delusion', 'increaser of pleasure', 'exciter of desire', 'cementer of friendship' etc.

However, he had been careful also to note that 'it is also well known for the tenacity of its fibre, which is employed by the mountaineers in Gurhwal and Sirmore for making a coarse sackcloth and strong ropes for crossing their rivers' and to note that 'it is remarkable that no one should yet have attempted to obtain it for commercial purposes, particularly as during the late war so many attempts were made to find an efficient substitute for this important plant'. Greville had ignored this information in compiling his entry on cannabis and chose instead simply to focus on what he saw as the 'vile' uses of the plant.

Indeed, doctors in India with less active religious convictions seem not to have paid as much attention to the intoxicating effects of cannabis preparations or indeed mentioned these in the context of the other uses of the plant. John Fleming, who was to become the president of the Bengal

[50] J. Royle, *Illustrations of the Botany and other Branches of the Natural History of the Himalayan Mountains and of the Flora of Cashmere* (Allen, London, 1839).

Medical Service during his time in Calcutta, published *A Catalogue of Indian Medicinal Plants and Drugs with their Names in the Hindustani and Sunscrit Languages* in 1810.[51] His entry on the plant made no mention of its use for intoxication and indeed seemed more concerned to dispute the idea that 'Indian ganja is a different species of cannabis from the cannabis sativa'. In 1833 George Playfair, a Superintending Surgeon in Bengal, translated an Indian *materia medica* called the 'Tareef Sereef' into English and this included a very positive assessment of hemp's medicinal uses and even a recipe for its preparation.

Take of Bidjia [bhang] 64 tolahs when the sun is in the division Sirtaam, white sugar 32 tolahs and pure honey 16 tolahs, cow's ghee 24 tolahs. First fry the Bidjia in the ghee, then add the honey in a boiling state, afterwards the sugar: use this in moderate doses daily and when it has been used for two months strength and intelligence will have become increased and every propensity of youth restored; the eye sight cleared, and all eruptions of the skin removed; it will prove an exemption from convulsions and debility and preserve the bowels at all times in a state or order. It will likewise give an additional zest for food.[52]

It was William Brooke O'Shaughnessy however who was to write the definitive account of cannabis of the early nineteenth century. While all of the above accounts written in India relied on earlier reports or at best referred to some personal enquiries and observations, O'Shaughnessy not only collected existing opinions but also conducted his own experiments with the drugs on both animals and humans. It does not seem surprising that it was O'Shaughnessy who was the first British doctor to decide to find out for himself exactly what the impact of cannabis substances was rather than to rely on hearsay or on recycled versions of other writers' compilations. He seems to have been a man of formidable energy and diverse interests and ended up being hailed as the saviour of the British Empire in India.

Born in Limerick in 1809, he graduated as an MD from Edinburgh University when only 21 and published his first research, a translation from the French of Lugol's *Effects of Iodine* in the following year. Just two years later he was on his way to India as an assistant-surgeon having impatiently answered 'certainly not' when asked on the application form for entry into the Indian Medical Service whether 'any person has received or is to receive

---

[51] J. Fleming, *A Catalogue of Indian Medicinal Plants and Drugs with their Names in the Hindustani and Sunscrit Languages* (Hindustani Press, Calcutta, 1810).

[52] G. Playfair, *The Taleef Sereef or Indian Materia Medica (translated from the original with additions)* (Medical and Physical Society of Calcutta, 1833).

any pecuniary consideration or anything convertible in any mode into a pecuniary benefit on account of your nomination?'[53] His nominee for service noted that 'I do hereby certify that . . . I received the said appointment for my friend William Brooke O'Shaughnessy through my gratuitous solicitation, his father being dead and his mother in ill health and that no money or other valuable consideration has been or is to be paid.'

On arrival in India he took on a number of projects. He eagerly conducted experiments with local drugs and medicines and published the results of these in journals such as the *Transactions of the Medical and Physical Society of Bengal*. Eventually he collected his conclusions and observations together in *The Bengal Dispensatory* and the *The Bengal Pharmacopeia* in 1842 and 1844.[54] In 1842 he also found time to publish *A Manual of Chemistry Arranged for Native, General and Medical Students*[55] and by then had been made a Professor of Chemistry and Medicine in the Medical College of Calcutta. He also seems to have taken on the role of an early criminal pathologist in his post as Chemical Examiner in Calcutta and wrote reports on poisoning cases in India that included the method that he had devised of detecting *lal chittra* in the body, the root used in India to cause abortion. He seemed to have a flair for this work, and indeed in a murder case in 1841 O'Shaughnessy found the critical piece of evidence, crusts of metallic arsenic in the stomach of the victim, despite the fact that the body that he worked on had been exhumed after being buried for eight months.[56]

His most famous role, for which he was knighted and through which it might be claimed that he saved the Indian Empire for the British, was as a pioneer of the telegraph system in India. As early as 1839 he had published the findings of his own experiments with electricity and the telegraph but at the time there was little interest in O'Shaughnessy's technology. With the appointment of a new Governor-General of India, Lord Dalhousie, in 1847 O'Shaughnessy's work was actively encouraged and by 1852 his results were so successful that the East India Company authorized immediate expenditure on lines to connect its major cities Calcutta, Agra, Bombay, Peshawar, and Madras. By 1856 he had overseen 4,000 miles of

[53] L/Mil/9/383/124 Assistant Surgeon's Papers.

[54] W. O'Shaughnessy, *The Bengal Dispensatory and Companion to the Pharmacopoeia* (Allen, London, 1842); *The Bengal Pharmacopoeia and General Conspectus of Medicinal Plants* (Bishops College Press, Calcutta, 1844).

[55] W. O'Shaughnessy, *A Manual of Chemistry Arranged for Native, General and Medical Students and the Subordinate Medical Department of the Service* (Ostell & Lepage, Calcutta, 1842).

[56] W. O'Shaughnessy, *Investigation of Cases of Poisoning* (Bishops College Press, Calcutta, 1841), 21.

cable laying and hanging as Director-General of Telegraphs in India. It was the rapid communication along these new wires of intelligence on enemy troop movements and tactics that was one of the key factors behind the successful British campaigns against the Indian rebels who fought the East India Company in 1857 and who almost destroyed British rule in Asia. Knighted in 1856 and retired in 1861, O'Shaughnessy managed to get through three wives and to live to the age of 80.[57]

Once his energies were focused on cannabis then the results were original and authoritative. In many ways they needed to be in order for cannabis medicines to be accepted by British doctors, given the often fierce prejudice against local medical systems on the part of many East India Company medical men. While it is true that some in India were prepared to try out the full range of Indian therapies—James Esdaile for example even experimented with mesmerism as a means of sedation during the 1840s using Indian hypnotists—a growing distrust towards the region's medical traditions and healthcare practitioners seems more common among the British medical establishment in India by the 1820s. For example, the first mention of the hemp plant and its properties in the *Lancet* came in 1829 as an aside in a larger diatribe by a British doctor in Bengal on the evils of Europeans using Indian wet-nurses when in Asia. As part of the attack on their efficiency that included such generalizations as 'their first object is to make money, their comfort is paramount and ingratitude is invariably expressed' came the accusation that they were 'persons, who generally eat opium and smoke a poisonous narcotic called *bhang*'.[58]

In 1842 O'Shaughnessy published the *Bengal Dispensatory and Companion to the Pharmacopoeia*. The section on cannabis spanned twenty-five pages and had already been partially published as 'On the Preparations of the Indian Hemp or Gunjah (Cannabis Indica)' in the *Transactions of the Medical and Physical Society of Bengal* of 1839. This was the most comprehensive assessment of the properties of cannabis preparations and of their effects as drugs and as medicines to appear by the hand of a British scientist in India during the entire period of colonial rule. It started with a frank acknowledgement of the drug's leisure uses 'the narcotic effects of hemp are popularly known in the south of Africa, South America, Turkey, Egypt, Asia Minor, India and the adjacent territories of the Malays, Burmese, and Siamese. In all

[57] For further details of O'Shaughnessy's career see J. Moon, 'Sir William Brooke O'Shaughnessy—the foundations of fluid therapy and the Indian telegraph service', *New England Journal of Medicine*, 276 (1967), 283–4.

[58] F. Corbyn, 'Management and Diseases of Infants under the Influence of the Climate of India' *Lancet* 2 (1828/9), 760.

these countries hemp is used in various forms by the dissipated and depraved, as the ready agent of a pleasing intoxication.' In the same paragraph however, O'Shaughnessy makes clear that 'in the popular medicine of these nations we find it extensively employed for a multitude of affections'. He was careful to balance his opening statement with a positive declaration of the beneficial uses of the plant.

Indeed, having observed the ritual of condemning narcotics and of giving a brief account of the plant's botanical characteristics and of the opinions on the drug of his predecessors, he settled to the real business of his entry. This was the 'several experiments which we have instituted on animals, with the view to ascertain its effects on the healthy system; and lastly, we submit an abstract of the clinical details of the treatment of several patients afflicted... in which a preparation of hemp was employed'. O'Shaughnessy had been experimenting on people, as well as on animals.

He was eager to defend this approach as he must have anticipated criticism. He was quick to point out that the various authorities that he had already summarized, a list that included Acosta, Royle, and Ainslie, had attested to the ability of hemp preparations to act as a stimulant for the digestion, as a sedative and as a painkiller. He then argued that 'as to the evil sequelae so unanimously dwelt on by all writers, these did not appear to us so numerous, so immediate or so formidable as many which have been clearly traced to over-indulgence in other powerful stimulants or narcotics, viz alcohol, opium or tobacco'. Having covered himself against detractors, he turned to his experiments.

It seems that his first subject in these tests was a 'middling sized dog'. Having been fed ten grains of Nepalese 'churrus' (charas) the hound 'became stupid and sleepy, dozing at intervals, starting up, wagging his tail as if extremely contented, he ate some food greedily, on being called to he staggered to and fro, and his face assumed a look of utter and helpless drunkenness'. It took him six hours to get over his little debauch. No doubt many dog owners would point out that the behaviour outlined above was very much what they would expect of their pet at the best of times so a smaller hound was procured and a larger dose administered. This dog was under the influence in fifteen minutes, 'in half an hour he had lost all power over the hinder extremities which were rather stiff but flexible; sensibility did not seem to be impaired and the circulation was natural. He readily acknowledged calls by an attempt to rise up.' It seems that O'Shaughnessy quickly became bored of canine subjects and turned his attention in time to most of the other corners of the animal kingdom.

It seems needless to dwell on the details of each experiment; suffice it to say that they led to one remarkable result—that while carnivorous animals and fish, dogs, cats, swine, vultures, crows and adjutants, invariably and speedily exhibited the intoxicating influence of the drug, the graminivorous, such as the horse, deer, monkey, goat, sheep and cow experienced but trivial effects from any dose we administered.

This extensive set of trials, which must have gained O'Shaughnessy a splendid reputation as an eccentric, encouraged him to turn his attention to humans. It seems that O'Shaughnessy was not the only eccentric involved in the trials. One patient who was suffering from severe rheumatism, two hours after a grain of cannabis resin in solution had been swallowed was reported as 'becoming very talkative, was singing songs, calling loudly for an extra supply of food, and declaring himself in perfect health'. Four hours later he was fast asleep and on examination was found to be in a state of catalepsy, which O'Shaughnessy discovered when 'on lifting up the patient's arm ... we found that it remained in the posture in which we placed it'. O'Shaughnessy found this response to the drug so fascinating that he could not resist playing with the unconscious patient, 'we raised him to a sitting position, and placed his arms and limbs in every imaginable attitude'. More seriously, attempts to revive him convinced the watching doctor that the drugs had acted as a sedative and as a painkiller. Once awake, the patient declared himself to be much improved and he was discharged three days later.

The experiment was repeated and had similar results. One rheumatic old coolie was given a dose of hemp in a little spirit and in no time at all 'became talkative and musical, told several stories, and sang songs to a circle of highly delighted auditors, ate the dinners of two persons subscribed for him in the ward, sought also for other luxuries we can scarcely venture to allude to, and finally fell soundly asleep'. It seems that in seeking for these 'other luxuries' the old coolie was hoping that the doctor would find him a girlfriend as well as giving him dinner and getting him drunk. Next day the patient 'begged hard for a repetition of the medicine, in this he was indulged for a few days and then discharged'. All of the cases of rheumatism that were experimented on were similarly relieved and O'Shaughnessy was quick to note that there were no side effects of headache or sickness.

A case of rabies was treated with cannabis doses and while it did not cure the disease, it allowed the patient constant relief from the horrendous hydrophobia of the condition to the extent that he could drink water, eat fruit, and swallow rice. O'Shaughnessy included this example as he was impressed by the power of hemp to alleviate the hydrophobia and he observed that if he could not cure, it was the duty of the doctor to 'strew the path to the tomb with flowers'. Cholera was also in town at the time of his experiments although O'Shaughnessy admitted that it seemed to be a mild strain of the disease. Cannabis tincture was administered to victims and it seemed to have the effect of controlling diarrhoea and vomiting and of inducing rest. O'Shaughnessy stressed in a footnote that he had experimented on European sufferers as well as on Indian patients and had seen excellent effects on both.

Tetanus was successfully treated with cannabis in the hospital and the lives of Chunoo Syce and Huroo were saved as was that of the man who turned up at hospital with 'a sloughing sore of the scrotum'. From O'Shaughnessy's account it seems that he was not the only British medical officer using cannabis in tetanus cases and he names Drs O'Brien, Esdaile, and MacRae along with the vets Hughes, Templer, and Sawyer as advocates of using the substance on humans and horses. It seems that at this time in Bengal British doctors were increasingly turning to cannabis as a remedy for tetanus.

A case of 'infantile convulsions' was treated with cannabis, and although the child was at one point 'in a sinking state' it survived not only the illness but a range of treatments that included 'two leeches ... to the head', 'a few doses of calomel and chalk', and a mouthful of opiates. The child was either very ill or it knew what was good for it as in one day it consumed 130 drops of cannabis tincture, the equivalent of fifteen times that given to the rheumatic who fell asleep so soundly that his body could be set into poses. O'Shaughnessy also treated delirium tremens with the drug, and found that considerable improvement could be effected through the administration of cannabis preparations.

The account of the cannabis experiments given by O'Shaughnessy suggests that the period of his trials of the drug was a merry time indeed, with drunken animals in and out of the premises and patients involuntarily uttering the odd 'loud peal of laughter', while medical students voluntarily tested the drugs on themselves, no doubt all in the name of science. 'Several pupils commenced experiments on themselves, to ascertain the effects of the drug. In all, the state of the pulse was noted before taking a dose, and subsequently the effects were observed by two pupils of much intelligence. The result of several trials was, that in as small doses as the quarter of a grain, the pulse was increased in fullness and frequency; the surface of the body glowed; the appetite became extraordinary; vivid ideas crowded the mind; unusual loquacity occurred; and with scarcely any exception great aphrodisia was experienced.' The effects of the cannabis drugs on the wards were such that even the dying could contribute to the unusual hospital atmosphere, one fading Hakim dreamily speaking 'in raptures of the inmates of his zenana and his anxiety to be with them'. Subsequent enquiry proved that the old man had never had such a collection of women, but the drug seemed to be helping him to an end that was veiled in the fantasies of pleasure.

O'Shaughnessy was convinced. He recorded in his 1839 paper that 'the results seem to me to warrant our anticipating from its more extensive and impartial use no inconsiderable addition to the resources of the physician'. Indeed, in his subsequent guide to the Bengal Pharmacopoeia of 1844 he described it as a 'powerful and valuable remedy in hydrophobia, tetanus, cholera and many convulsive disorders'[59] and as 'narcotic, stimulant and anti-convulsive, given in cholera, delirium tremens, tetanus and other convulsive diseases, also in neuralgia, in tic doloroux etc.'. He outlined the treatment to be used and advocated twenty minims and upwards, administered in syrup. He even helpfully included the recipe for the tincture of hemp: 'ganja tops two pounds, rectified spirit one gallon. Macerate for two days, then boil for twenty minutes in a distilling apparatus, strain while hot'.[60]

It is as necessary to be wary of O'Shaughnessy's conclusions as it is to investigate those of his less enthusiastic predecessors like Ainslie. While the latter had moral and religious convictions that meant that he would be immediately suspicious of anything that was taken simply to intoxicate, the former was an ambitious and entrepreneurial scientist from relatively humble origins who was evidently casting around for the means to establish a reputation and some degree of financial security. He was to achieve both through his work with electricity and the telegraph, but cannabis would have seemed a good prospect at one time. After all, this was a period when fortunes could be made from medical innovation, as Edward Jenner had demonstrated with his smallpox vaccine. It was also a time when opium made drug companies very wealthy as a painkiller and soporific in the preparations that satisfied Victorian Britain's appetite for patent medicines and tonics. His excitement about cannabis may not simply therefore have had scientific origins.

Nevertheless, it remained the case that an Honorary Fellow of the Royal Medico-Botanical Society of London and a Professor of Chemistry and

[59] W. O'Shaughnessy, *Bengal Pharmacopoeia*, 91.
[60] Ibid. 428.

Medicine had conducted extensive experiments and trials of hemp drugs.
As the chapter has shown, before these experiments and trials the drugs
were little known in Britain. Non-medical men mainly concerned themselves with hemp as a source of rope rather than as a source of medicine or
intoxication. British doctors and scientists relied on medical textbooks that
contained second-hand information gleaned not from personal experience
but from a quick glance along the bookshelves. Even the reports written by
East India Company doctors in India in the early nineteenth century suggested that their information was taken from asking around rather than
from direct contact with cannabis drugs and close observation of their
effects. O'Shaughnessy was therefore the first British medical man to conduct his own trials and to speak from his own varied and extensive experience. History shows that when he did speak, it was to say that cannabis
was a wonder-drug.

3

'From the old records of the Ganja Supervisor's Office': Smuggling, Trade and Taxation in Nineteenth-Century British India

CONSUMING CANNABIS IN INDIA

By the nineteenth century India was established as the main source of information for the British about the hemp plant and about medicinal and intoxicating preparations made from it. Yet hemp in India was not simply the source of information about cannabis substances for the British. It was also a source of income. The British were, after all, in India to make money. Before 1858 the British in India were employees of the East India Company that had traded spices, agricultural products, and luxury goods for profit since the seventeenth century. It had become militarized in the eighteenth century through wars with the French in India and because there was money to be made from hiring out soldiers as mercenaries to feuding local princes. As such, by 1757 its armies began to dominate large parts of India, and the company discovered that there was money to be made through taxation rather than trade. Dominating a region with an army means controlling its trading systems so taxation becomes both possible and profitable. By 1833 the East India Company had given up its old function as a trading company altogether and derived its profits solely from its role as an adminstration in charge of taxation.

Because the British were in India to make money, and because they were there to make money through tax, it is not in the least bit surprising to find out that they sought profits from the cannabis habits of India. Here was a government after all that had encouraged the Chinese to take up opium smoking so as to reverse the balance of trade that had traditionally existed between Europe and China and that had persuaded peasants all over Bengal to devote their land to growing poppies.[1] Not that Indians needed to be encouraged to take to ganja, bhang, and charas as hemp for narcotics had been extensively cultivated in South Asia and consumed widely in the region for centuries and indeed by the nineteenth century there were no signs of this changing. The British were the rulers of the world's largest producer of, and market for, cannabis narcotics and they decided to profit from it.

Not everybody in India used cannabis narcotics or indeed approved of them. One British officer could write in the 1840s that in Gurhwal 'the Khussea and the Doom class as above stated, alone cultivate the Hemp— the Rajpoots and Brahmins considering it quite a degradation to have anything to say to its culture and I am told that both in Kumaon as well as here it is reckoned a term of severe reproach and abuse for one of the latter class to be told that he cultivates it or that it is found close to his own door'.[2] Use in this part of India was evidently frowned upon by the elites of the area (Rajputs and Brahmins are of high status in the Hindu caste system whereas the Khussea and Doms are of lower status). Other reports also give the impression that use of the substances was limited only to certain classes of people in India. George Watt was a reporter on economic products for the Government of India and described in the 1880s his experience of users among the population in Bengal.

It must not be forgotten that the agricultural classes who of course constitute the vast majority of the inhabitants of India never partake of hemp narcotics. It is the artisans, mendicants and domestic servants who are the chief consumers; the middle and upper classes partake of hemp only at certain religious observances and even then to but a very small extent.[3]

[1] For a more detailed discussion of the opium trade see M. Emdad-ul Haq, *Drugs in South Asia: From the Opium Trade to the Present Day* (Palgrave, London, 2000); M. Booth, *Opium: A History* (Simon & Schuster, London, 1996); C. Trocki, *Opium, Empire and the Global Political Economy* (Routledge, London, 1999).
[2] 'Report on Hemp Cultivation etc in British Gurhwal by Captain H. Huddleston 14th July 1840', in *Papers Regarding the Cultivation of Hemp in India* (Agra Secunda Orphan Press, 1855), p. xviii.
[3] G. Watt, *Hemp or Cannabis Sativa (being an enlargement of the article in the 'Dictionary of Economic Products of India')* (Calcutta, 1887), 26.

However, the picture elsewhere seems to suggest that consumption was common to Indians in urban and rural contexts and throughout the many castes and classes. In Delhi it was observed that

both the rich and the poor among Hindus indulge in this narcotic, whereas only the lower class of Muhammedans partake of it. The habitual indulgers are to be found in saises, dhobis, faquirs, labourers, kahars, and halalkhors. They may be found in groups of 20 or 30 from three to five in the afternoon in the Kerdun Shuraf, Panch Kua, Eed Ghar or on the banks of the Jumna, clubbing together for a smoke at from a dumrie to a pic or two a head. The pipe is passed round until they become merry or angry and too often quite intoxicated.

Brahmins, mahajuns, and bunyas generally smoke charas at their own houses every day in the afternoon.[4]

Elsewhere in the country similar groups seem to have taken hemp narcotics. As in Delhi where workers like the saises (grooms and riders) and the labourers resorted to the drug, it was felt in Hyderabad that 'these drugs are taken by the labouring poor as a means to lighten their daily work'[5] and in the Central Provinces it was reported that 'persons whose employment subjects them to great exertions and fatigues, such as palki bearers etc. are solely enabled to perform the wonderful feats that they not unfrequently do by being supported and rendered insensible to fatigue by ganja'.[6] The working population of India resorted to narcotic preparations to combat the effects of a hard life and to aid rest and recovery or as one British official wrote, 'to dull the pain of exposure and starvation and ... to induce a pleasant languor and stupor'.[7]

Hemp narcotics also had a place in the religious life of Indian society. The faquirs are mentioned above as smoking it in Delhi while in the Bombay presidency it was noticed that 'ganja appears to be chiefly used by "gossavees", "faquirs" and other mendicants, generally of a low class'[8] and in Bengal it was considered an act of charity to supply religious wanderers with ganja.[9] Preparations of the drug were also used by the wider society within their religious and cultural rituals. In Hyderabad 'some people,

---

[4] J. Penny, Civil Surgeon Delhi, to Government of Punjab, in Papers Relating to the Consumption of Ganja and Other Drugs in India, *British Parliamentary Papers*, 66 (Hansard, London, 1891), 14.

[5] J. Stubbs, Commissioner Hyderabad, to Resident Hyderabad, ibid. 23.

[6] L. Neill, Sec. to Chief Commissioner, to Dept. Agriculture, Revenue and Commerce, ibid. 11.

[7] A. Rogers, Revenue Commissioner, to Government of Bombay, ibid. 59.

[8] L. Reid, Commissioner of Customs Bombay, to Government of Bombay, ibid. 54.

[9] Hem Chunder Kerr, 'Report of the Cultivation of and Trade in Ganja in Bengal', ibid. 141.

except Marwaris, offer it first to their gods'[10] and in Uttar Pradesh it was
noticed that 'there is also a concoction of bhang and sweetmeats called
majum, which is an accompaniment at festivals and other great gatherings
of the brethren'.[11] One such festival was that of the goddess Durgá, which
was celebrated with most energy in Bengal. There, drinks prepared with
hemp narcotics were integral to the celebrations, 'on the last day of the
Durgá Pujá it is religiously offered to every guest and member of the family,
and those who do not like to take it put a drop of it on their tongue by way
of acceptance'.[12]

It is also evident that it was not just the wealthier and elite groups who
lived in Delhi who used the narcotics and it seems that members of high-
income or high-status groups elsewhere in India were also consumers. In
Bombay it was asserted that 'all classes of the community make use of
hemp, and all castes of Hindus from the Brahmin downwards'.[13] In
Madras the elites seemed to prefer to drink their hemp preparations, 'bhang
is used in the shape of a drink prepared in various ways and chiefly
consumed by the better classes'.[14]

Indeed, one reporter despaired of any generalization when it came to
Indians and their favourite intoxicants.

It must always be borne in mind that a statement which holds good for any given
tract may be in no sense true of the tract next to it ... Thus there are certain tracts
which may be described as country-spirit consuming tracts, and others which may
be respectively described as opium, ganja and pachwai (rice/grain beer) consuming tracts; and it will be shown in the course of this report that not only is country-
spirit the main excisable article used in the tracts first mentioned, but that its
consumption elsewhere is comparatively unimportant. Similar statements hold
good of the opium, ganja and pachwai tracts. But when the various parts of each
of these tracts are examined in detail, all sorts of differences are found. In one part
of the country-spirit tract for instance there is a considerable consumption of tari, in
another pachwai is much used by certain classes, in some parts ganja is greatly
consumed and in other parts opium.[15]

In short, the picture that emerged from across India during the nineteenth century was of a population that enjoyed its intoxicants. These were

---

[10] Iajoodeen Hoosain, 'Report on the Subject of Ganja and Bhang', ibid. 26.
[11] 'Abstract of Replies Regarding Abuse of Ganja and Bhang [in Oudh]', ibid. 45.
[12] H. C. Kerr, 'Report of Ganja', ibid. 105.
[13] H. Carter, 'Memorandum on Effects of Hemp', ibid. 57.
[14] E. G. Balfour, Inspector-General of Hospitals, to Government of Madras, ibid. 80.
[15] *Report of the Commission Appointed by the Government of Bengal to Enquire into the Excise of Country
Spirit in Bengal 1883–84* (Bengal Secretariat Press, Calcutta, 1884), 4.

resorted to for the pleasure of stimulation or for the relief of torpor. They
were taken as aphrodisiacs by some and to enable a hard afternoon's work
by others. The elites in some parts of the country enjoyed them as much as
the workers did in the towns and in similar ways to that of the peasants in
the villages. The various classes and castes of the Indian population constituted the largest market in the world for cannabis products. The question
remains however, of how they were feeding their habits.

CULTIVATING HEMP AND MANUFACTURING 'GANJA'

Although found wild across India, the hemp plant which was cultivated
for the production of narcotics had certain specific environmental requirements. The soil was preferably a light sandy loam (called *poli* in Bengal),
able to maintain moisture and situated in a region where water was accessible and controllable throughout the winter as irrigation of the crop took
place at least twice between November and January. In other words,
the regional eco-system needed to have been capable of retaining water from
the monsoon until the beginning of the following calendar year, but should
not have been regularly susceptible to rains in the period from October to
March. Showers in late September or October killed the newly transplanted
seedlings. Prolonged rain in December and January disrupted the flowering
of the female plants as it encouraged new shoots that weakened the budding
flowers and also created conditions for the growth of *hírkati* or *sidlepoka*,
insects which attacked the plants. Strong winds at any time of the plant's
growth were thought to kill off the plants and certainly threatened to uproot
them.

  These requirements meant that the plants were cultivated only in certain
regions of India. By the 1870s the crop was known to be produced at
Sholapore, Ahmednugger and Khandeish in what is now Maharashtra,
at Vizagapatam, Salem, Tanjore, Madura, Nellore, Arcot, Coimbatore,
Kurnaul, Bellary (Tamil Nadu and Andhra Pradesh) and across Uttar
Pradesh in districts around towns such as Bareilly, Gorakhpur, and
Moradabad. In Bengal the crop was grown in the Ganja Mahal, a tract of
land straddling the districts of Bogra, Dinagepore, and Rajshahye which
totalled about 60,000 acres. Hem Chunder Kerr, a deputy tax collector
working for the British colonial administration, was sent on special duty to
the Ganja Mahal in 1876. His job was to survey the cannabis growing
district as the Board of Revenue of the Lower Provinces of Bengal had
realized that it knew so little about the ways in which such a lucrative

agricultural crop was prepared and brought to market. His account of the system remains the most complete and detailed set of insights into a cannabis producing economy available to the modern historian and the outline below relies heavily on his report.[16]

From this report it seems that Indian hemp was only one in the range that made up the local agricultural producer's portfolio of crops. In any one field, ganja was sown once every four years. It was reaped in March and the field was turned over to the cultivation of jute which was planted in May and harvested in October and which was closely followed by mustard which was harvested in February. Other crops raised from the field in the interval between hemp yields included potato, turmeric, tobacco, early rice, and ginger. In other words cultivated hemp was deeply embedded in the farmer's planning in the Ganja Mahal as it was included in both the annual crop production cycle and in the longer-term strategies of land use rotation systems.

The production of the crop was an intensive process involving large inputs of labour and also significant levels of land management. The first step was regular ploughing of the soil to be planted with hemp. This usually began in March or April, and between four and eight ploughings of the area were made at intervals of three or four days, the number of ploughings made depending on the condition of the soil and also on the means of the cultivator. By the end of April or the beginning of May, fresh earth was added to the ploughed area from surrounding ditches or nearby low land, a process called *bhorákátá*, and the margins around the field were weeded and these weeds added to the cultivated area as manure. The weeded borders were then raised by the addition of earth from ditches to form a barrier about 9 inches high around the cultivated area, a process called the *pagárbándhá*. If cow dung was to be added, it was put on the fields at this stage, before the monsoon season.

Throughout the four months of the monsoon season the land was continually ploughed and harrowed with a bamboo 'ladder' called a *moi*, the objective being to circulate the water into the soil and to prevent it from sticking into clods. As Hem Chunder Kerr remarked, 'the belief is that the oftener the land is ploughed, the better is the crop'.[17] As the rains became less regular in September cow dung and household refuse, which had been stored throughout the year as compost, were added to the field and allowed to sit on the surface for about ten days. After this the field was

---

[16] Kerr, 'Report of Ganja', 94–154.   [17] Ibid. 109.

again ploughed about eight times while it was harrowed with the *moi* after every two ploughings.

The field was now finally divided into ridges, called *shulis*, into which the seedlings would be transplanted. These ridges were raised on top of the field and were about 18 inches broad at the base and about 3 feet apart from one another. The distance between these ridges could differ considerably from plot to plot, determined by the economic arrangements of the cultivator. If he had arranged simply to grow the crop for a wholesaler who would send in labourers to reap and prepare the hemp, the cultivator would reduce the space between ridges so as to 'present a closely planted field to the eyes of the purchasers'.[18] If the cultivator was going to harvest and prepare the crop within his household he would leave a larger distance between the ridges so that the effort involved in getting into the fields to maintain the plants and to harvest them was rendered less time consuming.

The seedlings (*púl*) were placed about 8 inches apart in these ridges some time in the middle of September. By this time they were four or five weeks old and between 6 and 8 inches high, having been grown in a nursery bed since the first two weeks of August. This nursery was always in the lightest loam available in the village and was often shared between individual cultivators where such soil was not easy to find. The nursery was preferably near to the dwelling of the cultivator or cultivators so as to make guarding the seedlings against birds easier to accomplish as part of the daily routines of the household. Plots where *muthá* (*Cyprus rotundus*) grew naturally were favoured as this grass-like vegetable was thought to be evidence of dry soil. The land had been regularly ploughed before acting as a nursery, it was furrowed before planting so as to manage rainfall if it came, and grass was allowed to grow in amongst the seedlings as it was believed that it protected them from wind damage.

These ridges survived for about six weeks, and by the end of October had been gently weeded and then dismantled, the earth directly around the roots remaining in place while the spare earth was kept on one side. Manure, of oil cake or of oil cake and cow dung combined, was then placed around the piles of earth at the foot of the plants, which was all that remained of the ridges, care being taken to place the manure in position so as not to cover the delicate plants with it. The spare earth on one side was then used to remake the ridges over the manure. The field's ridges were dismantled and remade over a number of days as the whole process for each

[18] Ibid. 111.

ridge had to be completed in the same day in order to prevent the spare soil drying out.

A couple of weeks later the plants themselves were attended to as the lower shoots were removed to encourage upward growth. The area between the ridges was ploughed and furrowed and the ridges again manured and earthed over, which increased their size by about 3 inches. The agricultural machinery for the ploughing and furrowing was specially made for the purpose and the animals used to pull it were specifically selected for the job: 'the ladder used for this purpose is made of the proper size to suit the width of the trenches ... the ploughs too are small, with short yokes, and the bullocks used are of small bulk [and] specially trained to the work, for the bullocks have to walk between the rows of plants and unless trained for the purpose they are apt to injure the plants'.[19]

By now it was time for the 'ganja-doctor'. Locally called the *poddár* or *parakdár*, which was translated as the 'ganja-doctor' by Hem Chunder Kerr, this specialist arrived in late November. His main task was to identify the male plants by examining the filaments or stipules of the crop and to destroy them. It was only parts of the unfertilized female plant that were useful in the production of the intoxicating preparations and as such it was vital that the males of the crop were weeded out before pollination could begin. He made three or four inspections over the end of November and the start of December, snapping the offending males to identify them so that once his inspection was completed the cultivator could go into the field to remove the broken plants. The skills of the *poddár* determined the success or failure of the crop

the *poddár* is an indispensable person in the ganja business and the result of the cultivation depends mainly on his care and diligence in weeding out the male plants; for ... the presence of a few *mádi* plants, or correctly speaking of male plants in the field suffices to injure the entire crop inasmuch as all the plants run into seed, and the ganja yielded by them is very inferior and scarcely saleable.[20]

After the 'ganja-doctor' had completed his rounds the cultivator devoted his attention to the remaining plants safe in the knowledge that they had a right to be in his field. He continued to trim lower stems to encourage upward growth and transplanted some remaining plants to parts of the ridges where there were now gaps after the weeding out of the males. After these transplantations the ridges were once again dismantled, manured, and rebuilt for a final time. A first irrigation of the soil would have taken place

[19] Kerr, 'Report of Ganja', 112.   [20] Ibid.

after the initial inspections of the fields in early December and a second watering took place at the end of the month or at the beginning of January, care being taken to soak the land but not to immerse it.

Finally the female plants began to sprout flowers in January and over the next month these matured to the state where they were heavy in the sought-after resin. Once the flowering tops of the plants turned yellowy brown and the heavier leaves fell off the crop was ready to be harvested and the 'ganja' manufactured. This took place over the month between the middle of February and the middle of March. At this point the cultivator could sell the crop to a wholesaler who would employ his own men to harvest the plants and manufacture the drugs. Alternatively the cultivator may have opted to harvest and prepare the crop himself.

If the latter was the case then a *chátor* was prepared. This was a space of ground for the manufacture of the ganja that was usually a paddy field, selected because it was flat. It was cleared of all weeds and stubble and huts were erected around it for those who were going to work on and watch over the crop. The plants, by now around 5 feet tall, were cut about 6 inches from the ground, gathered together in bundles of 50 or 60, and carried to the *chátor*. Here the bundles of flowering heads were placed under mats and trampled, new bundles being regularly added to the developing mushy mass of flowers, this process continuing over four days. The constant trampling was necessary as 'the compacted mass is kept under pressure for some time to promote chemical changes'.[21] In some areas it was thought that rolling the flowers was more effective than trampling them. The trampled variety was called 'flat ganja' and the rolled variety was sold as 'round ganja'. The former was associated with the Bombay region and the latter with Bengal[22] although the evidence suggests that in Bengal both types were produced.[23] Fragments of the flowering tops that had broken off from the main layers of ganja were gathered together and sold under the name *chúr* ganja. This product was held to be more potent than round or flat ganja as it contained only flower heads and their resin and none of the other parts of the plant which inevitably got mixed in during the process of making round or flat ganja.

Quite simply then, the whole process of cultivating hemp for narcotics and manufacturing the ganja products shaped the ecology and society of the areas in which it was an important part of the economy. As has been demonstrated, land was carefully managed through the processes of

[21] R. Chopra, *Chopra's Indigenous Drugs of India* (UN Dhur, Calcutta, 1958), 88.
[22] Ibid.
[23] Kerr, 'Report of Ganja', 116–20.

ploughing, manuring, and irrigation and the soil was doctored to prepare it
for the hemp crop. Hydro-management systems were devised to preserve and
make accessible the water in the eco-system. Where wells were available a
complex of narrow irrigation channels was dug in the fields and water was
raised using a bamboo lever, at the one end of which was a basket for the
water and at the other end of which was a counterweight to lift the basket
from the well when full. Where the water table could not be relied upon
tanks were constructed near the fields to capture and keep rainwater and this
was then distributed by hand. Trees were removed so as to ensure that no
shade fell on the crop as the plants needed constant exposure to sunlight to
develop the resin in the leaves. Farm land was set aside for the nursery and
for the *chátor*, the area of manufacture, and these plots also needed specific
preparation where the consistency and content of the soil and the ground
was worked on to change it from its natural state to a cultured one.

    While the ecological environment was significantly altered by the pro-
cesses of hemp cultivation and ganja preparation, life itself was also affected
in important ways for the cannabis cultivator. Indeed, as a valuable source of
external income and as a labour intensive crop, hemp could often dominate
the lives of its producers. Hem Chunder Kerr noted that of all the crops
grown in a year by local agricultural producers it was hemp that most
affected the cultural cycle of the cultivator's year. Although the cultivators
were a mix of Hindus and Muslims in the Ganja Mahal, all celebrated
weddings at the same time: 'the weddings in the families are, as a rule,
celebrated in the months of Jeyt, Assár and Srában, when the sale of the drug
is over and when they have paid out of the proceeds thereof the zemindar's
rent'.[24] The hemp then was the source of the cash with which land rent
was paid, in other words it was the source of access to land in the first place
and the other crops mentioned earlier were grown for subsistence or supplementary income. Indeed not only does Hem Chunder Kerr's statement
suggest that hemp production affected the timing of cultural activities like
marriage, it also seems to have been the source of funds to pay for these
festivals. Little wonder then that, 'before the trampling commences the
persons to be so employed salute the ganja before placing their feet on it',[25]
a ritual that Hem Chunder Kerr described in pointing out that 'the trampl-
ers invariably make a bow to the ganja before they place their feet on it'.[26]
Indeed, the different religious communities were careful to apply their astro-

    [24] Kerr, 'Report of Ganja', 123.
    [25] G. Watt, *A Dictionary of the Economic Products of India*, vol. ii (Calcutta, 1889), 113.
    [26] Kerr, 'Report of Ganja', 116.

logical traditions to the production processes such was the significance of the crop. Hem Chunder Kerr reports that

Among the Hindu cultivators it is not usual to commence the cutting in the afternoon of a Thursday, or on any particularly unlucky day. Among the Muhammadans the sowing, the transplantation and the reaping must all commence on a Friday which in their opinion is a lucky and holy day.[27]

While hemp production lay entangled with the peasant producer's cultural activities it also influenced his social encounters. The range of processes described above meant the introduction of a host of outsiders into the life of the village. Gangs of labourers from the neighbouring districts of Purneah and Dinagepore would appear in the area in April to be employed in the initial stages of the production process of ploughing the land ready for transplantation. Later on, workers would arrive from Jessore, which had formerly been a ganja producing area and it remained a skills reservoir to be tapped into by cultivators and producers. The 'ganja-doctors' were traditionally from that area although by the time of Hem Chunder Kerr's report there was evidence that their skills had been picked up by local men as well. Workers from Jessore were also employed in the production processes, in the trampling of the flowering heads and also in the tying of the bundles of ganja, which was an important step as waste material in the bundles would still be weighed and charged duty on.

Then there were the wholesale buyers of the drug. There were two varieties of these buyers. First there were those that came and purchased the crop in the field and who intended to have their own men reap the hemp and process it. Then there were those that simply came to purchase the prepared ganja made by the cultivators themselves. The latter group of buyers often did their dealings using regional brokers that dealt with the producers of the drug through a network of local agents. The former group of buyers, however, was far more closely involved in the rural areas, arriving in the villages themselves in January, inspecting fields, and negotiating directly with the peasants. They could fix a price for the estimated ganja yield of a crop while it was still in the field and would then allow the cultivators to go ahead and process the crop on the promise of delivering it over for the agreed sum once the ganja was manufactured. Alternatively, they made cash advances to the peasants to secure rights to the field and sent in their own teams of coolies to process the crop. The ganja was subsequently never removed all at one go but was left stored in the areas of

---

[27] Ibid. 115.

manufacture and delivered in instalments according to variations in the market price of the drug.

This meant that the involvement of the wholesalers in the villages did not simply come in the form of a brief annual visit. Rather the relationship between the wholesaler and the cultivator/producer over one crop went on for much of the subsequent year. This was especially so as it was apparent that 'the *goladars*' [wholesalers'] agents resort to all kinds of tricks'[28] to avoid prompt payment or indeed to avoid payment at all. This would result in cultivators having to go after their money, which could often involve extensive travel, Hem Chunder Kerr citing 'an instance in which the poor cultivator had to go to the purchaser's house, hundreds of miles away from Nowgong, for his money and had to come back with only a portion of the sum owing to him'. The wholesalers that bought from the Ganja Mahal were based all over what is now West Bengal and Bihar in cities such as Calcutta, Patna, and Bhagalpur and they in turn sold on to dealers that supplied markets as far away as modern day Pakistan, Trinidad, and even London.[29]

TAXATION, ILLICIT PRODUCTION, AND THE SMUGGLERS

With markets for the drugs spread across India and throughout the Indian population, and with large regions such as the Ganja Mahal dedicated to supplying these markets, the British were unable to resist the temptation of siphoning taxes from such an extensive trade. Between 1793 and the 1850s the East India Company officers were happy just to derive a steady income from the commerce in cannabis and were not concerned to intervene too directly. The system that they devised demanded that the retailer of the drug, before approaching the peasant producers, had to turn up at the office of the local colonial official and pay for a licence that would grant him permission to proceed and buy his stock of the drugs. Having done this, he was free to head on to meet his supplier and to purchase as much as wanted, after which he was equally free to go and sell it wherever he wanted. In other words, the government was simply concerned to guarantee that the licences

[28] Kerr, 'Report of Ganja', 132.
[29] Ibid. 138. See Chapter 4 for the medical market for cannabis in London and Chapter 7 for the market in the West Indies among Indian migrant workers.

were being bought and they cared little about how much of the drugs were being produced or consumed.[30]

It was decided by the middle of the century that there was more money to be had from the trade as the scheme was changed in 1854 and the system in operation by the time of Hem Chunder Kerr's report was to tax the wholesaler in his place of business rather than at the point of purchase or production. In other words once the stock of 'ganja' was in the wholesaler's warehouse the district collector there would be able to assess his approximate holdings and to maintain surveillance of how much the retail buyers were taking from the wholesaler. The amount sold by the wholesaler to the retailer was therefore taxed.

The key to the success of levying this duty was an accurate knowledge of the amount of 'ganja' in the system. To this end the British had introduced a series of licences under Act II of 1876. The peasant producer of the hemp plant had to approach the authorities to obtain a licence to cultivate the crop. This was intended to inform the district collector which peasants in his area of supervision were producing hemp so that he might keep these people under surveillance. He employed an establishment specifically for this purpose in Nowgong, the town that was the district headquarters of the Ganja Mahal. Among the duties of this staff were regular tours of the area so that they could form estimates of the area under cultivation and watch the progress and health of the crop, thereby supplying approximations of how much ganja might reasonably be expected to come onto the market in February and March. When the crop was ready and the ganja had been processed, the cultivator (or the wholesaler who had purchased the standing crop and prepared it with his own staff) applied for a licence to store the drug. To be granted this licence he stated how much of the drug he intended to store and the permit was made out to cover this amount.

The wholesaler meanwhile had gained a permit to export the crop from the Ganja Mahal back to his home district where he intended to sell the ganja to retailers. This permit, completed by the district collector of his home district, stipulated how much of the drug he could legally take back with him. He also had a licence to buy the drug once in the Ganja Mahal and to comply with the requirements of this licence he needed to present his purchases to the supervisor of the staff employed to look after the district's ganja trade. Here his stock of the drug was weighed and checked against

[30] This summary is taken from G. Rainy, *Report on the Manufacture and Smuggling of Ganja* (Bengal Secretariat Press, Calcutta, 1904), 9.

the amount that he was allowed to import back into his home district. Once all was in order the wholesaler's carts or boats were searched to make sure that he was not smuggling. With this completed the authorized bales, each marked with an excise stamp, were loaded and the wholesaler headed for home with his stocks.

While this was the system as the British intended it to operate it does not necessarily follow that this was how it did operate. It is possible to trace in the historical records a number of ways in which the ganja trade took on the British government's attempts to have a slice of their profits. The cannabis cultivators were one group that began to find ways around the British system. They combined the sheer extent of the suitable land available to them to grow hemp on with what appears to be an awareness of the limitations of the colonial state. The establishments set up by the British to supervise the ganja trade were expected to have a working estimate of how much hemp was being grown in any one year. They were supposed to gain this estimate through pursuing what one collector called their 'outdoor enquiries', which involved walking around the villages and arriving at approximations of the scale of hemp cultivation by observation and by taking information from the cultivators themselves. Hem Chunder Kerr quickly discovered, on ordering a measurement of the fields, that there was a considerable difference between the area that the cultivators were declaring as set aside for hemp and the area that was actually made up of plots of the crop.

No one on behalf of Government surveyed the fields and there was nothing to prove that the area alleged was really what was under cultivation. The difference between the reported area (2113 bigás and 2 cottás) last year and the actual (3111 bigás 9 cottás) found by measurement showed a difference of 998 bigás and 7 cottás . . . this would amount to an annual loss of revenue to the extent of Rs 478 852. There is nothing to show that there has not been a similar disparity between the total of the reported area and the actual under cultivation in former years; on the contrary, the presumption is strong that there was marked disparity.[31]

Quite simply the cultivators knew that the representatives of the colonial state were too few in number to accurately and regularly assess the large areas devoted to hemp cultivation and indeed that those representatives were dependent upon them for information. As Hem Chunder Kerr recorded, an independent assessment was impossible as 'the supervisor has not the means of making such an inquiry, as he has not men enough to go to the *chators*, or to the houses of about 200 men'.[32] Indeed it was a prominent feature of the recommendations of Hem Chunder Kerr's report that consid-

[31] Kerr, 'Report of Ganja', 143.   [32] Ibid. 121.

erable alterations should be made to the staff of the ganja supervisor's office, including mounted police to increase patrols of the Ganja Mahal and the stationing of officers of the supervisor's establishment every 16 square miles.

They will find no difficulty from June to September to measure every inch of the fields proposed to be devoted to hemp and submit a report to the collectorate. After transplantation it will be devoted to hemp and submit a report to the collectorate. After transplantation it will be their duty to visit the fields from time to time and see how the cultivation is progressing and submit progress reports. In December and January they should prepare an estimate of the probable yield of each field. The work during the manufacturing season will be heavy; it will then be their duty to visit the chátors frequently, to take note of the quantity daily manufactured, and to see that the produce is regularly and promptly forwarded to store houses.[33]

These elaborate expansions of the ganja supervisor's responsibilites were designed to overcome one of the main peasant strategies of resisting the colonial state's determination to tax the ganja trade. This was to declare that a certain amount of land was being cultivated, so as to appease the state's representatives and so as not to arouse the suspicion of the authorities which would not believe that no hemp was being produced at all. However the peasant producers then brought supplementary, undeclared areas under cultivation for hemp. It is little wonder then that Hem Chunder Kerr noticed activity on the peripheries of the area that he was surveying: 'in the northern and western parts of the Ganja Mahal there are jungles which the people are gradually clearing and bringing under cultivation'.[34]

The cultivators also used the layout of their farms so as to make sure that the state's representatives had no way of knowing how much ganja had actually been made from the hemp crop. The manufactured crop was not gathered together in one warehouse or barn but was deliberately spread around the various buildings and lean-tos erected across the farmer's land. Consider the observations on storage in the report:

During my stay at Nowgong I took the supervisor with me and visited several places used for the storage of ganja. I found it stored at every convenient nook or corner, without any care or guard. I saw a quantity of flat ganja kept in a cowshed situated in an open place and without any doors in the house of one Fakir Bakhsh. In one Piru Mandal's place I found some hemp lying in an open verandah of a room in the house. In the homestead of one Chhedor Mandal there was a large quantity of round ganja lying in an open hall of the house on planks placed on the floor. I also saw some flat hemp in an open room and inside a cowshed in the house of a respectable ryot [smallholder] named Kukur Sardár.[35]

---

[33] Ibid. 146.   [34] Ibid. 122.   [35] Ibid. 121.

The objective of this was to make the job of the state's representatives almost impossible as even if a visit was made by the supervisor or one of the staff of the ganja establishment he would not be able to accurately assess the amount of the drug that had been produced. Hem Chunder Kerr was well aware of this as he wrote, 'there is nothing to prevent the concealment of a portion of what has been prepared or to prevent some of it being taken away secretly at night, before the supervisor or his chuprasees visit the khullian. If the ryot has stored the prepared produce, the supervisor can examine "the store", he cannot search the several houses of the cultivator.'[36] Fire was also woven into the ways in which the producers of ganja eluded colonial attempts to tax them accurately. The heat and dryness of that part of Bihar and West Bengal from March to July and the ad hoc storage facilities meant that 'accidental' fire provided an ideal story to cover for anomalies in ganja stocks. The report despaired that

Even of the quantity reported a good portion might disappear without any let or hindrance. Fires are frequent, and reports frequently sent in of quantities of the drug having been destroyed thereby. An open shed or cowhouse where ganja is stored is of little value. Ten rupees suffice to replace one, and yet a couple of bales burnt in it is equal to a duty of over Rs. 212. There is nothing to prevent the removal and sale of the drug and the subsequent firing of the hut to cover the nefarious transaction. Every such transaction would amount to a clear gain of nearly Rs. 200.[37]

While the cannabis cultivator made sure that the state was in the dark about how much of the drug was available, a network of smugglers developed to carry undeclared produce from the region. The Government of India feared that the river system of Bengal favoured the illicit export of drugs, especially as 'the river Jabuna runs through the ganja tracts; it is navigable all the year and smugglers have every opportunity for taking away ganja of any description with very little risk of detection'.[38] As such Hem Chunder Kerr suggested a system designed to combat this, 'to prevent smuggling from the houses of the cultivators'.[39] This involved a guard boat on the river Jabuna and 'a preventive station at Sahebgunge on the Atraie river' as these waterways provided the ideal means of removing illicitly produced hemp narcotics from the area without having to pass along the roads which were patrolled by the colonial police and which passed through the towns of the district administrators.

Evidence of this smuggling trade was of course difficult to come by because of the secretive nature of the processes involved and only rarely

[36] Kerr, 'Report of Ganja', 144. [37] Ibid. 145. [38] Ibid. 144.

could the colonial officers boast that 'three men were seized by the police with one seer and a half of round hemp and sent in for trial. They were subsequently convicted at Beauleah.'[40] More often than not, the authorities only caught elusive glimpses of the smugglers going about their business.

In December following, a couple of police constables and a village watchman belonging to thana Manda in Rajshahye were, about 9pm on their way to Bálihar, when they saw two persons crossing the field with something on their heads. On their shouting out, the men dropped their loads and ran off. It was then found that they had dropped 36½ *kutcha* seers of flat hemp. The drug was taken possession of by the constables but the culprits were never traced.[41]

Sometimes it was even possible to get hints of those cultivators that were involved but it was impossible to prove any allegations. 'In the first week of January last two men were seized with seven tolás of round ganja at the Táherpore Haut. Their defence was that they had received them from a ganja grower, who however denied having ever given it to the men, who were found guilty of the offence and punished.' In this example there is every reason for the cultivator to deny knowledge of the smugglers' claim. He could be prosecuted for participating in the illegal trade, he had no doubt already received payment, and the colonial state had no means of proving that the crop was his.

Overall then, Indians involved in the ganja trade found a host of ways of frustrating the colonial state's attempt to squeeze revenue from them. Cultivators exploited the limitations of the state to accurately measure the amount of hemp that they were growing by not declaring honestly how much they were producing on their land and by cultivating previously unused land out of the sight of colonial officers. Once the ganja was grown and processed they also came up with ways of concealing the true extent of their stocks. They did this first of all by making use of the opportunities for hiding the manufactured drugs presented by the extensive spaces available to them on their land. As such they deliberately spread their holdings of the narcotic across the full extent of their farms so as to prevent accurate assessment of their stocks. They also exploited the fact that fire was a common hazard in the glare of the long, hot summers, and quantities of the drug which had already disappeared into smuggling networks were passed off as lost in blazes that were in fact far from accidental. Finally, the cultivators worked with the wholesalers of the drugs and made use of the river systems of their region as a transportation system to send illicit supplies out from the Ganja Mahal and into smuggling networks designed to get the

[39] Ibid. 146.   [40] Ibid. 142.   [41] Kerr, 'Report of Ganja'.

narcotics to the markets without the state being able to exact its toll on them.

THE WILD PLANT AND WILD DRUGS

It seems that the revenue systems described above, the most sophisticated developed by the 1870s to deal with the taxation of the cannabis trade in India, were insufficient to overcome the problem of illicit production and smuggling of the drugs. These systems were instituted by the government of Bengal, although it seems that the other regional administrations in India were less concerned with accurate taxes on the trade.

Bombay and the North-Western Provinces were said to be two of the three largest areas of consumption in India and yet they had failed to pay much attention to the issue of taxation. These governments contented themselves with a tax-farming system whereby licences to sell cannabis products were auctioned off every year to the highest bidders. They kept no record of what was produced or consumed, or indeed what prices were being charged for preparations of hemp. They simply received the annual fee for the licences and forgot about the subject. In Assam and the Central Provinces there were more concerted efforts to tax the ganja trade. In the Central Provinces it seems that the producers were compelled to store their produce in government warehouses (*golas*) once the hemp was gathered from the fields and had been manufactured into intoxicating substances. When the wholesalers had done their deals with the producers the government released the agreed amount of the drugs from the warehouse but only once the appropriate duty had been paid. In Assam, there was a large market for the drugs among the coolie population working there on the tea plantations (it is interesting to reflect on the fact that the British were ensuring a supply of one drug to Indians to guarantee that they worked hard enough to provide the Englishman with a cheap cup of his favourite stimulant). The British in Assam imported quality ganja from Bengal and supervised the sale of it to the tea-workers through agents that had paid the government for licences and who had to sell from government warehouses. The close control of the trade, in an area where natural conditions encouraged the wild growth of hemp, meant that there were deemed to be problems of covert production and smuggling.

The hemp plant (cannabis sativa) grows in a wild or rather naturalised condition in most districts of the Assam valley and of Cachar. From this source a small amount of illicit trade proceeds, chiefly in bhang; but this seems to be of very little importance for while the plant grows profusely it is generally reported not to secrete in its leaves the narcotic principle to any great extent. The reports are rather conflicting in this respect however and it would seem according to some writers that a considerable quantity is annually brought into Assam by the hill tribes beyond the frontier.[42]

This issue of the wild plant and its preparations was also a problem in Bengal. While the production of ganja necessitated cultivated hemp, other preparations of hemp used by peasant consumers did not. *Siddhi*, *patti*, and *sabji* were all words for the leaves, or were sometimes used to describe preparations of the leaves, of the wild hemp plant. Hemp grew naturally all over India and in certain parts of the country it was noted that 'the plant is so plentiful as to be extensively used as bedding for cattle'.[43] It certainly grew wild in the Ganja Mahal area, Hem Chunder Kerr pointing out that in fact 'it grows in almost every district of Bengal and Behar [*sic*]'.[44] The leaves of this wild strain of hemp could be washed and ground into a paste which was then diluted with water and mixed with a range of spices that included aniseed, rose leaves, or black pepper to be drunk as a 'refreshing draught'.[45] Alternatively, the leaves could be boiled with a little oil which caused them to yield their resin in the form of a jelly-like substance on the surface of the water. This jelly was then mixed with dried milk and syrup and baked over a fire into tablets called *májun* or *májum*. Alternatively the leaves could be ground into a powder and used in a range of foods, such as *barsh*, a north Indian conserve enjoyed by Muslim consumers.

While properly prepared, cultivated ganja was the preferred narcotic, it was the case that the local environment could provide alternative, albeit inferior, hemp drugs. The state's levies on ganja could therefore be resisted by turning to other, perhaps less satisfactory, but more freely available forms of narcotic. Hem Chunder Kerr realized this in his report, stating that 'there is a longing for intoxicating substances in human nature which nothing can eradicate, and those who will be obliged to forgo ganja on account of high duty will replace it by bhang, charas, daturá, arrack and other stuffs'.[46] Bhang preparations were often prepared in the houschold from locally gathered plants, one writer noting that for this reason it would be difficult for the colonial state to control their use: 'It would be impracticable to hold a man responsible for the existence of a wild plant growing within a certain radius of his hut, and it would be impossible to prohibit

---

[42] Watt, *Hemp or Cannabis Sativa*, 27. The summary above is taken from this account.
[43] Watt, *Dictionary*, 118.   [44] Kerr, 'Report of Ganja', 152.
[45] Ibid. 105.   [46] Ibid. 148.

him gathering, from such a plant, the daily quantity used by himself and his family.'[47]

However there was also a retail trade in preparations made from the wild plant that were manufactured for urban markets. As such, producers in the Ganja Mahal, who were on the whole occupied with cultivated hemp for ganja, were careful to set aside plots to the wild strain which could grow with little attention on marginal soils. Bhang retailers then paid the farmers for access to these plots of wild hemp and sent in their own labourers to cut the crop and to bring it back to their shops where it was prepared. Interestingly, Hem Chunder Kerr produces figures for the amount of wild cannabis removed from one district near Monghyr in the Ganja Mahal. It shows that during the 1870s the amount of the wild plant produced and exported by the Ganja Mahal had steadily increased, from 1,721 maunds in 1873, to 2,824 the following year, which was a peak as it then levelled out at around 2,300 maunds in 1875 and 1876 (a maund weighed the equivalent of about 82 imperial pounds).[48] It seems to be no coincidence that this was the period when the troublesome licence system for cultivated ganja outlined above was introduced. This was also the time when the duty on flat ganja was raised from two rupees to almost three rupees per seer and when duty on *chúr* (the fragments left over from the ganja manufacturing process) increased to four rupees per seer. In other words there is plenty of evidence that many Indians simply switched their consumption patterns to resist the taxes of the British. These figures also show that the cannabis cultivators were using the wild plant to maintain income and to resist the administration's attempts to cut into their revenues.

CANNABIS AND THE CRIMINAL CONNECTION

> The only safeguard against illicit trade in excisable articles is constant and unwearied vigilance.[49]

To summarize then, the British in India were the rulers of the world's largest market for cannabis products while at the same time they were governing the largest system for producing the varieties of drug to feed that demand. Throughout the nineteenth century they chose to tax this trade so as to guarantee themselves a share of the profits to be had from Indian hemp habits.

[47] Watt, *Dictionary*, 117.   [48] H. C. Kerr, 'Report of Ganja', 152.
[49] Ibid. 143.

This was indeed a lucrative trade to be taking a slice of, as one reporter by the 1880s could point out that tax in Bengal alone on cannabis was worth almost Rs 200,000 which meant that the trade that it was derived from must be worth more than £500,000 a year. This did not take into account the illegal trade in the substances. This made tax on cannabis in Bengal a more important source of revenue than tax on opium sold in the region.[50]

Indians, however, were far from being passive in the face of the British determination to take larger and larger amounts of cash from the cannabis drugs trade. Where taxes meant that ganja was too expensive, Indians could grow wild hemp and manufacture inferior but less expensive drugs from this. However, Indians also took to an illegal trade in ganja to escape the demands of the colonial state. Cultivators grew undeclared crops, lied to the colonial officials about their output, and concealed supplies in isolated barns to await shipment. Smugglers came from the wholesalers by night and, under cover of darkness, whistled the hidden drugs away over the fields and onto boats where the illicit hoard would float past sleeping guard posts and down the rivers to the cities of the empire.

Because of this economic battle between the British and the cannabis trade cannabis came to take on criminal associations in the minds of colonial officials. As the British had devised a number of regulations to guarantee their income from the trade, a refusal to cooperate with revenue raising measures was not simply a financial offence but a criminal one. Cultivators and wholesalers seeking simply to maintain their income became criminals and their trade became a subject of suspicion even where little could be proved: 'in dealing with an article so highly taxed as ganja, it would be an unwarrantable demand on human credulity to expect that the mere fact of a paucity of detection and conviction would justify the belief that illicit trade in the article was limited,' reasoned Hem Chunder Kerr[51] and a British colleague, the Collector of Rajshahye agreed, grumbling that 'non-seizure of Ganja is no indication of the non-existence of smuggling'.[52]

There may have been a wariness of cannabis products in the minds of certain British writers in the eighteenth and nineteenth centuries that was based on a general condemnation of all things intoxicating and William O'Shaughnessy's experiments had done much to dispel many of these misgivings. But as the nineteenth century wore on cannabis drugs became a matter for the 'constant and unwearied vigilance' of India's police establishments and as such took on an air of criminality. This was entirely the

[50] Watt, *Hemp or Cannabis Sativa*, 21.   [51] Kerr, 'Report of Ganja', 143.
[52] Ibid. 142.

creation of the British system. The colonial government attempted to raise more and more revenue from a trade that had been established long before they arrived and by doing this suddenly turned into criminals those cultivators and traders that simply acted to protect their profits. By the 1870s, cannabis was taking on criminal associations in the minds of the British in the empire. This was at just the same time, as the next chapter will show, that it was increasingly believed to be the cause of a sinister and lurking madness in the Indian population as a whole.

4

'The Sikh who killed the Reverend was a known bhang drinker': Medicine, Murder, and Madness in Mid-century

THE SISTER OF SLEEP

In the thirty years after William O'Shaughnessy's experiments in Calcutta attitudes towards cannabis began to sharpen across the British scientific community. In Britain itself cannabis medicines enjoyed some popularity among doctors who were inspired by O'Shaughnessy's work and who happily conducted their own experiments on themselves and their patients. However, in the empire British officers gathered evidence that convinced the Government of India that there was a direct link between cannabis use and mental illness. This, together with the connection that was becoming established in many official minds in that country between crime and hemp preparations that was discussed in the previous chapter, meant that the British in India began to view cannabis with grave suspicion and to go as far as to consider ways of prohibiting its use in the country. This chapter will explore these decades of contrasting opinions among British doctors and administrators around the world and will examine the evidence that many of them produced in support of their assertion that cannabis use led to insanity. It will demonstrate that this evidence was in fact deeply flawed.

The *Provincial Medical and Surgical Journal* of 1842 shows how British doctors had been immediately enthused by the work of William O'Shaughnessy in India. Doctor W. Ley reported 'On the Efficacy of

Indian Hemp in some Convulsive Disorders' and directly referred to O'Shaughnessy, recommending 'the use of the resin of the garden hemp as a narcotic and antispasmodic'. Ley used it in a case of a woman with 'spinal disease' who could barely sleep for spasms and pains in her back and who had spent much of the previous five years confined to a waterbed. She experienced instant relief, slept for twelve hours, and found herself able to straighten her limbs. He repeated the experiment on a number of cases that included an injured shipwright, a noisy infant, a swollen teenager, and a coachman whose 'bursa was as large as a small pot orange' and in all of them found hemp useful. He concluded that he had 'the most perfect confidence in the power of the remedy to produce relaxation of the muscles, heavy sleep, and during its action abatement of pain' although he did point out that one of his patients complained that 'he did not think it did his head any good at all'.[1] Evidently impressed by this report the editors of the *Provincial Medical and Surgical Journal* invited O'Shaughnessy to revise and update his original findings published in the *Transactions of the Medical Society of Calcutta*. They serialized it in January and February of 1843, devoting the front pages of both editions to his work on Indian hemp.[2] Indeed, O'Shaughnessy wrote a separate letter to the *Journal* to recommend hemp for its 'extraordinary anticonvulsive power'.[3]

Following this, the *Journal* reported a meeting of the Royal Medico-Botanical Society over which Earl Stanhope presided and for which 'the meeting room of the society was exceedingly crowded throughout the evening, the gentlemen present manifesting the most lively interest in the discussion'. Ley read a paper on hemp and O'Shaughnessy, on leave from India, also presented on the subject. It was pointed out by Ley that 'there is an old act of Henry the Eighth yet in force by which it [hemp] is forbidden to be soaked in ponds or running streams where cattle drink. The older writers speak of it as a violent poison and state that the water in which it has been soaked produces its effects almost as soon as drank.' However both he and O'Shaughnessy, who was presented with the diploma of a corresponding member of the society at the meeting, confirmed that 'hemp is of value in the treatment of spasmodic diseases'. Indeed, the evening revealed that there was an enthusiasm for experiment with hemp drugs on the part of other British doctors.

---

[1] W. Ley, 'On the Efficacy of Indian Hemp in some Convulsive Disorders', *Provincial Medical and Surgical Journal* 4 (1842), 407–9.

[2] *Provincial Medical and Surgical Journal* 5 (1842–3), 343, 363.

[3] Ibid. 397.

Dr Copland said that he had obtained specimens of the drug some time since from Savory's, and had tried it both medicinally and physiologically ... he took thirty drops of the tincture and shortly experienced a slight acceleration of the pulse with slight giddiness and exhilaration of spirits; in an hour or two he felt an inclination to sleep. The next day he took sixty drops with increased effect, attended with dryness of the fauces [*sic*]; the day after the dose was one hundred drops when there was an increase of the giddiness and he slept soundly. The pulse all this while was not increased above six or seven beats in the minute. He had tried it in disease; he had given it to an hysterical female complaining of sleeplessness; with her it had produced giddiness and slight nausea, but she slept soundly.[4]

O'Shaughnessy's work had an immediate impact on British medical practice and it continued to exert an influence over the following decades. Throughout the subsequent years the British medical press monitored the growing debate about the use of cannabis drugs. One area of medicine in which doctors seemed especially concerned to experiment with them was in the treatment of women. In 1847 the *Provincial Medical and Surgical Journal* carried an article by Benjamin Barrow that reported his use of cannabis drugs in period pains. He had treated the patient in the past, 'a married lady, twenty-six years of age, of a thin spare habit [and] of a naturally feeble constitution', by using large doses of opium or morphine that had simply caused her to vomit. Aware of O'Shaughnessy's work and prompted by a friend to try the drug he resorted to the tincture of cannabis indica. His treatment had a dramatic impact: 'the extremities and body became cold, and when I saw her she was perfectly pulseless, the eyes wide open and staring, the pupils somewhat contracted and quite insensible to the strongest light'.[5] A couple of years later the same journal reported the use of cannabis preparations by a Dr Churchill in his treatment of a variety of health problems in women that included controlling a threatened miscarriage and stopping bleeding from uterine cancer.[6] He found it extremely useful in all instances and reported none of the side effects outlined in 1847.

The *Provincial Medical and Surgical Journal* was the predecessor of the *British Medical Journal* and in the first volume to be published under this new title in the 1850s a letter from a doctor in Darlington showed that the *Journal* and its contributors continued to have a lively interest in Indian hemp in the treatment of females. Called to the bedside of Mrs——,

---

[4] 'Royal Medico-Botanical Society February 22 1843', ibid. 436–8.

[5] B. Barrow, 'A Case of Dysmenorrhoea in which the Tincture of Cannabis Indica was Employed with some Observations upon that Drug', *Provincial Medical and Surgical Journal* (1847), 123.

[6] 'General Retrospect', *Provincial Medical and Surgical Journal* (1849), 333.

Doctor Jackson found that she was threatening to go into a premature labour in only the seventh month of pregnancy. This had happened with four previous pregnancies, so Jackson decided that he wanted to stop the contractions altogether. Tincture of Indian hemp was administered and resulted in 'giddiness in the head, stiffness of the tongue, difficulty of articulation, a tingling sensation all over the body, especially in the tips of the fingers, severe vomiting with eructations every five minutes' and indeed he records that 'such being the symptoms at my second visit I was afraid that my patient was about to "quit this mortal coil" '. Next morning, however, the symptoms had abated and the treatment had been successful as she progressed to the ninth month of pregnancy, when she gave birth to a healthy child.[7] Oddly however, cannabis drugs had been recommended earlier in the 1850s as a means of stimulating rather than delaying delivery during pregnancy. It was reported in the *Edinburgh Monthly Journal of Medical Science* in July 1850 that 'parturient action seemed to be very markedly and directly increased after the exhibition of the hemp'.[8] In exploring the possibilities of cannabis preparations in labour it seems that British doctors were rather belatedly catching up with their colleagues elsewhere in the world. It has been argued of cannabis that in China 5,000 years ago 'it was particularly prized for its ability to relieve labour pain, speed up delivery and reduce post-delivery bleeding ... traces of cannabis were identified in the remains of a young girl who died near Jerusalem in the fourth century AD. Scientists have deduced that she was in all probability given the drug to ease the pains of childbirth. This has been one of the most ubiquitous historical applications.'[9]

Indeed, the *Edinburgh Medical Journal* continued to publish in this period articles on the range of uses that were being found for cannabis. In 1858 it reported a story from Honduras where Staff Assistant-Surgeon E. W. Skues had successfully treated a 9-year-old girl for tetanus by administering the drug so that 'the child was kept almost constantly narcotized'. She fully regained use of the afflicted arm after twelve days.[10] In 1865 the journal reported a case of traumatic tetanus being treated by the use of cannabis in India. The Professor of Surgery there, J. Fayrer, told how he gave the Indian labourer, whose body was rigid with the condition,

[7]   T. Jackson, 'Uncertain Action of Cannabis Indica', *British Medical Journal* (1857), 15.

[8]   J. Simpson, *The Obstetric Memoirs and Contributions of James Simpson* (Black, Edinburgh, 1855), 374.

[9]   P. Robson, *Forbidden Drugs* (Oxford University Press, Oxford, 1999), 66.

[10]   E. Skues, 'Tetanus Treated with Extract of Indian Hemp', *Edinburgh Medical Journal*, 3 (1858), 878.

'a bazaar preparation of opium made for opium smokers' while also dosing him with Indian hemp and chloroform. The man recovered and was able to walk home.[11] In 1869 the vice-president of the Medico-Chirurgical Society of Edinburgh published his account of the use of Indian hemp in Chorea.[12] He argued that 'the value of Indian hemp as a therapeutic agent is well established, but a singular difficulty has been experienced in securing for it the confidence to which it is evidently entitled'. He realized that this was because 'we are apt to be deterred from the use of a remedy by such pictures of its more peculiar actions as are given of the abuse of the drug in countries where it is resorted to as a means of intoxication and of its action in the cases of patients who under its use became tortured by ocular illusions and spectres of horrible form'. However, the outcome of the cases of chorea spasm that he treated were so successful that he recommended cannabis medicines to all who were attempting to control spasms and even related a case that he had read of in America where the drug had been administered to control hiccups that had tortured a patient for five days.

Indeed, by the 1870s cannabis was being used to treat insanity. At the Sussex County Lunatic Asylum at Haywards Heath there seems to have been something of a taste for experiment with all sorts of techniques for the treatment of mental illness. Among the approaches tried out, for example, was electricity, which was very much in the trial and error stage of development at the time.[13] When applied to the patients it had all manner of impacts. Some patients seemed to exhibit an improvement in their state of mental awareness and the superintendent could report of a farmer's daughter that 'electricity has lately been employed, since when she has appeared brighter and less inclined to suicidal attempts. Both the patient and her friends acknowledge the benefit that has resulted from the use of the electric treatment. She converses rationally, employs herself in needlework skilfully, is, in fact, now convalescent and leaves the Asylum shortly.'[14] Others, however, seemed greatly upset by the electrocution: one patient 'was excited when first placed under its influence and required to be restrained by four nurses'. The risks that such a violent and unknown regime could entail did not seem to worry the medical staff despite the often

[11] J. Fayrer, 'A Case of Traumatic Tetanus Treated by Opium Smoking and Internal Administration of Chloroform and Hemp', *Edinburgh Medical Journal*, 10 (1865), 716.

[12] D. Douglas, 'On the Use of Indian Hemp in Chorea', *Edinburgh Medical Journal*, 14 (1869), 777–84.

[13] A. Beveridge and E. Renvoize, 'Electricity: A History of its Use in the Treatment of Mental Illness in Britain during the Second Half of the Nineteenth Century', *British Journal of Psychiatry*, 153 (1988).

[14] S. Williams, *Sussex County Lunatic Asylum, Fourteenth Annual Reports for the Year 1872* (Bacon, Lewes, 1873), 40.

serious physical injuries caused by their experiments: 'the number of cells [batteries] was from 20 to 24; occasionally this number had to be reduced as there was a tendency to cause charring of the skin'.[15]

With a medical staff willing to try out unknown therapies on their patients it is little wonder that cannabis was also used in the asylum's therapeutic strategy. In detailing the range of chemicals that had been used in the hospital the asylum superintendent, a Mr S. Williams, presented the following example: 'Case II Eighteen years of age. Mania, supposed to have been caused by fever. Treated with bromide of potassium and Indian hemp, which, having no perceptible effects, were omitted after nine days' trial and morphia and hydrocyanic acid substituted. Recovered in 122 days after admission.'[16] More common at the asylum, however, was the use of cannabis preparations to treat migraine. Williams produced his report of the trials of cannabis drugs with migraine sufferers in the *Practitioner* in November 1872 as he was entirely convinced by its efficacy in tackling the condition, arguing that 'several years ago we were induced to make a trial of the Indian hemp and have since used it frequently and have nearly always seen it productive of more or less benefit to the patient'. He also showed an awareness of the misgivings of many of his colleagues about the side effects of the drug as he was careful to point out that 'this drug may be taken for very many months in comparatively large doses, without producing any unpleasant side effects or in any way injuriously affecting the economy. It would also seem that, unlike opium and some other narcotics, it may be given up abruptly without requiring the exercise of any fortitude by the patient.'[17]

The use of cannabis drugs in asylum medicine was most famously championed by Thomas Clouston, who won the Fothergillian Gold Medal of the Medical Society of London in 1870 for his work with them in the treatment of mental illness at the hospital that he was in charge of in Carlisle. The paper that he published in the *British and Foreign Medico-Chirurgical Review* in 1870 showed that he had been experimenting on his patients at the Cumberland and Westmorland Asylum with opium, bromide of potassium, and cannabis.[18] His formulation of the problem and his attempt to solve it was straightforward enough.

[15] S. Williams, *Sussex County Lunatic Asylum, Fourteenth Annual Reports for the Year 1872* (Bacon, Lewes), 44.

[16] Ibid. 17.   [17] Ibid. 45–7.

[18] T. S. Clouston, 'Observations and Experiments on the Use of Opium, Bromide of Potassium and Cannabis Indica in Insanity, Especially in Regard to the Effects of the Two Latter Together', *British and Foreign Medico-Chirurgical Review*, 46 (1870) and 47 (1871).

So many cases of insanity consist of simple brain excitement and in so many more is excitement the most distressing symptom that if we could discover any agent which would subdue this excitement and at the same time not interfere with the improved nutrition of the brain which rest, tonics and good diet will effect, and on which complete recovery of its normal functions depends, such an agent would be a most incalculable blessing.

He pointed out that medical studies of narcotics and stimulants tended to be made on patients that were 'free from excitement' and so he had decided to see what effects they may have on those who were in the agitated stages of their mental illness. He was careful to mention O'Shaughnessy's conclusions on cannabis in order to justify his including it in the list of substances given to the patients. While this included the drugs mentioned above, he also administered 'four ounces of a good Scotch whisky' and 'a pint of beef tea made from a pound of good beef' to the patients and indeed he was careful to ensure that no one missed out on the fun as both he and his assistant took a dose of each of the various treatments as well. He cheerfully admitted that there was no good scientific reason for this: 'curiosity alone prompted me to take the drugs myself', he wrote.

His results pointed to the usefulness of cannabis mixed with potassium of bromide. Of the twenty-six times that it was given it succeeded in subduing the excitement of the patient on each occasion, whereas opium only succeeded in nineteen of the cases, whisky in fourteen, and beef tea in none. Opium was the quickest to take effect while cannabis was slightly slower and, in a couple of instances, its power to sedate was preceded by a short increase in the agitation of the patient. Whisky was the most dangerous in respect of the latter effect as while it did eventually sedate its immediate impact was 'aggravation of the excitement ... so great and troublesome ... as to put it out of the question as a sedative for maniacal excitement'. Cannabis and potassium of bromide was also useful for bringing the patient's temperature under control and for stimulating the appetite.

Having observed the effects of single doses on patients he also subjected certain of his inmates to prolonged courses of the treatments. Over twelve weeks opium was administered three times daily to a group of patients in steadily increasing doses. After this length of time the treatment was discontinued until the same time the next year when he began to give them potassium of bromide and cannabis three times a day. His paper records that 'I found this treatment so beneficial to the patients that I have continued it now for about eight months with a few days' intermission occasionally in all the patients.' The excitement of the patients was allayed in all the examples and it continued to have this effect over the whole nine months in which it was given. Opium tended to lose its effects after a week or so. With the cannabis mixture, however, all the subjects gained weight, their bowels remained unaffected and even 'their tongues all remain clean'. Among the patients that he successfully treated were JP, a 27-year-old man that 'tore out all the windows of a gentleman's dining room' and who was made 'free from excitement' by cannabis and the bromide after opium and antimony had failed. EB, a 33-year-old woman who was 'violently mani-acal' after the birth of her fifth child, was treated with the cannabis and bromide compound every three hours and at the time of writing was considered 'almost well'. An 18-year-old lad, WB, who was 'incoherent, restless, violent and destructive' before treatment with the mixture was before long 'coherent and rational'. Clouston was convinced and wrote confidently that

if a mixture of potassium and Indian hemp so subdues intense excitement that when not taking this medicine the patient is noisy, violent, destructive, sleepless, and rapidly losing weight, and when taking it he is quiet, semi-rational, dresses and eats properly and remains in this state for six weeks till the disease in its natural course runs into its quiet stage, I think here we have a palliative of great value and importance.[19]

Henry Maudsley, the president of the Medico-Psychological Association and the Professor of Medical Jurisprudence at University College London, was quick to check Clouston's results. Referring to them in his presidential address to the annual meeting of the Association in 1871 he reported on his impressions of the usefulness of the Carlisle Superintendent's mixture of bromide of potassium and cannabis indica. His findings were equivocal. He seems to have been committed to the idea that a calm in the patient that was artificially induced was likely to be no such thing, as stupor was not the same as peace. As such he worried that 'chemical restraint' might be having no benefit whatsoever. However, he admitted at the end of his speech that 'I have treated a case of acute and violent mania in a man with cannabis Indica and bromide of potassium as recommended by Dr Clouston with the best possible results: he recovered in a week, when there was every possibility that the disease might have lasted for weeks or even longer.'[20]

---

[19] T. S. Clouston, 'Observations and Experiments on the Use of Opium, Bromide of Potassium and Cannabis Indica in Insanity, Especially in Regard to the Effects of the Two Latter Together', *British and Foreign Medico-Chirurgical Review*, 205.

[20] H. Maudsley, 'Insanity and its Treatment', *Journal of Mental Science*, 17 (1871–2), 334.

The idea that this relationship between madness and cannabis could be reversed and that use of the drug induced rather than cured mental illness was also being explored during the middle decades of the nineteenth century. The most remarkable exposition of the idea that cannabis could cause madness in this period was made by Mordecai Cubitt Cooke, a teacher turned curator at the India Museum who was a founder of the Society of Amateur Botanists and who helped to popularize science in the Victorian imagination through his magazine *Science Gossip*. Best known for his studies of mushrooms that culminated in his eight-volume *Illustrations of British Fungi*, he received an honorary degree from Yale and was awarded the Victorian medal of honour by the Royal Horticultural Society.

While this information is easily found in his *Dictionary of National Biography* entry, there is no record there of his *The Seven Sisters of Sleep* published in 1860.[21] This book was dedicated as follows

To all Lovers of Tobacco, in all parts of the world, juvenile and senile, masculine and feminine, and to all abstainers, voluntary and involuntary

To all Opiophagi at home and abroad, whether experiencing the pleasures or pains of the seductive drug

To all haschischans, East and West, in whatever form they choose to woo the spirit of dreams

To all buyeros, Malayan or Chinese, whether their siri-boxes are full or empty

To all coqueros, white or swarthy, from the base to the summit of the mighty cordilleras

To all votaries of stramonium and henbane, highlander or lowlander,

And To all swallowers of Amanita, either in Siberia or Elsewhere

These pages come greeting with the best wishes of their obedient servant, The Author.

The book showed its author to be anything but a dull academic as it was riddled with classical allusions and translated fables. The volume was written as a celebration of, and a study in, sleep and of the intoxicants that were used around the world to induce rest where it would not come naturally: 'when care, or woe, or wan disease steals for a time the mortal from his allegiance to the calm and blue-eyed Sleep, then do the sisters ply their magic arts to win him back again, and by their soothing influence, lull him to rest once more and again unlock the portals of the palace of dreams'.[22]

[21] M. Cooke, *The Seven Sisters of Sleep: Popular History of the Seven Prevailing Narcotics of the World* (Blackwood, London, 1860).

[22] Ibid. 5.

On the subject of cannabis the book wove a web of fable and legend before offering a surprisingly frank assessment of its pleasures and perils. Cooke recounted a variation of the tales that surrounded the origin of the word assassin, commonly believed to be a corruption by the European Crusaders of the Arabic word 'hashashin' that referred to soldiers whose ferocity lay in cannabis intoxication.

A youth who was deemed worthy by his strength and resolution to be initiated into the Assyrian service was invited to the table and conversation of the grand master or grand prior; he was then intoxicated with henbane (hashish) and carried into the garden, which on awakening, he believed to be paradise. Everything around him, the houris in particular, contributed to confirm his delusion. After he had experienced as much of the pleasures of paradise—which the prophet has promised to the blessed—as his strength would admit, after quaffing enervating delight from the eyes of the houris and intoxicating wine from the glittering goblets, he sank into the lethargy produced by debility and the opiate, on awakening from which after a few hours, he again found himself by the side of his superior. The latter endeavoured to convince him that corporeally he had not left his side but that spiritually he had been wrapped into paradise and had then enjoyed a foretaste of the bliss which awaits the faithful, who devote their lives to the service of the faith and the obedience of their chief. Thus did these infatuated youths blindly dedicate themselves as the tools of murder, and eagerly sought an opportunity to sacrifice their terrestrial in order to become partakers of eternal life.[23]

In his assessment of the drug Cooke began by citing the work of O'Shaughnessy and of Moreau, the French psychiatrist who had experimented with 'hashish' in the 1840s and whose work will be examined in a little more detail below. He then painted a picture of the delights of cannabis intoxication.

A small dose seems only to influence the moral faculties giving to the intellectual powers greater vivacity and momentary vigour. A larger dose seems to awaken a new sensibility and call into action dormant capabilities of enjoyment. Not only is the imagination excited but an intensity of energy pervades all the passions and affections of the mind. Memory not only recurs with facility to the past but incorporates delusions with it, for with whatever accuracy the facts may be remembered they are painted with glowing colours and made sources of pleasure. The senses become instruments also of deception, the eye and the ear not only are alive to every impression, but they delude the reason and disturb the brain by the delusions to which they become subject. Gaiety, or a soothing melancholy, may be produced, as pleasant or disagreeable sights or sounds are presented.[24]

[23] M. Cooke, *The Seven Sisters of Sleep: Popular History of the Seven Prevailing Narcotics of the World* (Blackwood, London, 1860), 220.

[24] Ibid. 232.

However, he warned quickly that 'the incautious use of hemp is also noticed as leading to, or ending in, insanity, especially among young persons who try it for the first time'. He told stories of the hallucinations that users had experienced: Dr Moreau had found that 'a little hideous dwarf, clothed in the dress of the thirteenth century, haunted him for some time'. Another example, of an Arab cook who was 'addicted to the intoxicating hachisch', was given where the man had been haunted by a Turkish soldier who sat on the kitchen stairs and smoked a pipe, refusing to talk or to move. These hallucinations were the key to the problem for Cooke and he warned, 'These hallucinations seem to be manifested independently of any then existing affection of the brain and the individual appears under other circumstances fitted for the usual avocations of life. They may be only symptoms of a previously disordered intellect but they may also be the starting point from which insanity is developed. In all instances in which these hallucinations occur, watchfulness is necessary, since, in the majority of cases they terminate finally in derangement of the brain to the extent generally denominated madness.'[25]

Yet for all his concern to show that the use of hemp was implicated in mental illness, he was certainly not attacking the drug or siding with temperance campaigners. He opposed the suggestion that these drugs were harmful per se and forcefully argued that 'to talk of the degraded Chinese as barbarians indulging to an awful extent in opium and the ignorant Hindoo and Arab as in madness revelling in debauches of hemp confections is an evidence of the workings of the same narrow-minded prejudices under which some who abstain from alcoholic stimulants rail and rave at those whose feelings and habits lay in an opposite direction, charging upon the enjoyments of the many the excesses of the few.'[26] Mordecai Cooke was no instinctive killjoy then and was certainly no advocate of the stimulant-free or narcotic-free life. His book was one of the first to frankly recognize both the perils of cannabis and the potential of its pleasures and to carefully separate out the consequences of 'enjoyment' of the drug and 'excess' in it.[27]

Cooke had clearly been impressed by the work of the Frenchman Jacques-Joseph Moreau. He published *Hashish and Mental Illness* in 1845,

---

[25] Ibid. 241.

[26] Ibid. 229.

[27] The book is all the more remarkable in the balance of its tone when compared with the rash of publications in the USA after 1850 that were concerned to paint nightmare visions of cannabis use. See for example F. H. Ludlow, *The Hasheesh-Eater* (Harper, New York, 1857), who stated that 'I shall relate how ecstasy by degrees became daily more and more flecked with shadows of an

the result of a remarkable thesis and some brave experimentation. Moreau was an intriguing character indeed. The son of a French soldier who had distinguished himself in Napoleon's armies, Moreau was a successful medical student who chose the path of psychiatry under the tutelage of the famous French *aliéniste* Jean Étienne Dominique Esquirol, a man still considered to be one of the pioneers of modern western psychiatry. While accompanying a wealthy patient on a convalescent tour of North Africa he became aware of the use of cannabis in the form of hashish in Egypt. He took the drug and having experienced its possibilities became convinced that it had a use in nineteenth-century psychiatry.

He did not think that it caused mental illness. Neither was he particularly interested in its possibility as a treatment for insanity. Instead he saw it as a means of experiencing madness while still sane: 'I saw hashish, or rather its effect upon the mental faculties, a significant means of exploring the genesis of mental illness . . . hashish gives to whoever submits to its influence the power to study in himself the mental disorders that characterize insanity.'[28] He was sure that the use of cannabis would enable him as a scientist to take a journey into the realm of insanity while allowing him to retain his reason under the influence of the drug and to return to a fully sane state to record his observations once its effects had passed. His experiences were startling and often dramatic. For example, Moreau recounted the evening that followed the consumption of a dose before dinner: 'I took a spoon and stood en garde against a comptier of candied fruit with which I was preparing to duel . . . I suddenly ran my hands through my hair. I felt millions of insects eating my head. I sent for an obstetrician, who was then with Madam B. to have him deliver the female of one of the insects who was having birth pains and had chosen for her "bed of pain" the third hair from the left of my forehead. After a painful labour the animal brought into the world seven little creatures . . . I saw my child, my beloved son in a blue and silver sky. He had white wings trimmed with pink.'[29] But these were not the experiments of an aesthete or of a romantic, they were the tests of a nineteenth-century scientist eager for closer knowledge of the illnesses of the mind.

---

immeasurable pain' and that 'torture, save at rare intervals, swallowed up happiness altogether, without abating in the least the fascination of the habit', p. xiii; see also H. Kane, *Drugs that Enslave: The Opium, Morphine, Chloral and Hashisch Habits*, (Presley Blakiston, Philadelphia, 1881).

[28] J. J. Moreau *Hashish and Mental Illness*, trans. G. Barnett (Raven Press, New York, 1973), 15–17.

[29] Ibid. 8–9.

His conclusions were that 'everything leads us to believe that [the primary lesion] results from some disturbance, some change in the circulation' and he was convinced that mental illness was 'linked essentially to a completely organic and molecular change'.[30] He dismissed the existence of hallucinations, instead arguing that humans experienced hallucinatory states. As his interest was mental illness rather than cannabis the work carries less significant observations on the drug. He was sure that the mood of the individual was important in determining the response to hashish intoxication, and he compared its effects on the whole to being in a state of 'sleepless dream, where sleep and the waking state are mingled and confused'.[31] Enigmatically, he hinted at the start of the book of the dangerous allure of the drug once used repeatedly: 'at first curiosity led me to experiment upon myself with hashish. Later, I readily admit, it was difficult to repress the nagging memory of some of the sensations it revealed to me.'[32] It seems that the most radical medical trials involving cannabis of the century had a lasting impact on the scientist that had used himself as a guinea-pig, either through the lingering pangs of withdrawal or through the hauntings of hallucinations.

As the century progressed, the work of Moreau was noted within the British psychiatric establishment. For example, William Ireland wrote a speculative piece in 1878 in which he sought to explore the nature of thought without language. He wrote that 'the condition following the use of cannabis or Indian hemp, closely resembles the delirium of insanity', which is very different from asserting that the drug caused insanity and was much nearer the Frenchman's conclusions about cannabis. Ireland later noted that he had indeed read Moreau and observed that 'the magnifying influence following intoxication through cannabis upon the distance of visible objects is only a part of a general exaggeration of impressions, mental as well as sensual'.[33]

Such assessments of cannabis and its impact on mental functioning were increasingly rare by the 1870s, however. While writers like Moreau and Ireland were careful to emphasize that cannabis induced a state that was like madness, many others were becoming convinced of a more straightforward and direct relationship between cannabis and insanity. Indeed, those that asserted this more direct relationship could turn to compelling sets of evidence to justify their positions.

[30] Ibid. 205–8.   [31] Ibid. 19.   [32] Ibid. 15.
[33] W. Ireland, 'On Thought Without Words and the Relation of Words to Thought', *Journal of Mental Science*, 24 (1878), 431.

CANNABIS AND THE LUNATIC ASYLUMS OF INDIA

> There can, however, be no doubt that its habitual use does tend to produce insanity . . . of the cases of insanity produced by the excessive use of drugs or spirits, by far the largest number must be attributed to the abuse of hemp.[34]

In 1872 the Government of India issued the above statement at the end of a comprehensive review of cannabis consumption in the colony. This review had had the following remit.

It has been frequently alleged that the abuse of ganja produces insanity and other dangerous effects.

The information available in support of these allegations is avowedly imperfect, and it does not appear that the attention of the officers in charge of lunatic asylums has been systematically directed to ascertain the extent to which the use of the drug produces insanity.

But as it is desirable to make a complete and careful enquiry into the matter, the Governor-General in Council requests that Madras, Bombay etc. will be so good as to cause such investigations as are feasible to be carried out in regard to the effects of the use or abuse of the several preparations of hemp. The inquiry should not be simply medical but should include the alleged influence of ganja and bhang in exciting to violent crime.[35]

The survey went out to colonial officers across India, to magistrates, tax collectors, and policemen as well as to doctors and to scientists, and its conclusions were presented in 1872. On the one hand many showed a great distrust of hemp preparations—'Hushiarpur says that in March 1864 the Nehung Sikh who killed the Reverend Mr Janviers (missionary) was a known bhang drinker,'[36] asserted the Punjab authorities, while Hyderabad forwarded the opinion that 'it is generally said, and I believe with much truth, that when a man "runs amuck" or a female commits "suttee" that before committing the act they are intoxicated by the use of hemp in some form or other'.[37] Those in Berar were afraid that 'Bhang is also taken by immoral people as an "aphrodisiac" as tending to excite the sexual passions. Preparations of hemp are also much used by women for the purpose of procuring abortion,'[38] while an old medical officer serving in Burma was

---

[34] 'Papers Relating to the Consumption of Ganja and Other Drugs in India', *British Parliamentary Papers*, vol. 66 (Hansard, London, 1891), 92.
[35] Ibid. 7–8.   [36] Ibid. 17.   [37] Ibid. 29.   [38] Ibid. 27.

able to assert that 'most of the acts of Mutiny of 1857 were undertaken under the influence of bhang, charas or ganja'.[39]

However, it is just as clear that not all British administrators in India had negative opinions of cannabis or of cannabis users. It appears that many believed, as did those in the Central Provinces,

and apparently not without great show of reason, that persons whose employment subjects them to great exertions and fatigues, such as palki-bearers &c., are solely enabled to perform the wonderful feats that they not unfrequently do, by being supported and rendered insensible to fatigue by ganja; and the use of ganja leaves in them no after effect of an injurious kind.[40]

These officers had views of the hemp user that were opposed to those which regarded him as violent or lunatic. There were some, however, that had no opinion at all in so much as they were oblivious to the issue and unable to offer observations one way or the other on cannabis use and its effects. For example in the summary of reports in Bombay it was noted that 'most of the Superintendents of Jails write to say they have no experience as to the extent the abuse of ganja proves an incentive to crime, and few of them seem to have had their attention drawn to the subject'.[41]

There was, therefore, a lack of consensus among British administrators in India on the subject of cannabis and cannabis use in the 1870s. The vivid descriptions of the effects of cannabis and of the volatility of cannabis users outlined above might therefore be dismissed as the moral panic of a minority of officials which was certainly not uniformly shared in the British administration. Yet the resolution of the Government of India at the end of the cannabis inquiry was quite clear that 'it does not appear to the Governor-General in Council to be specifically proved that hemp incites to crime more than other drugs or than spirits. And there is some evidence to show that on rare occasions this drug, usually so noxious, may be usefully taken. There can, however, be no doubt that its habitual use does tend to produce insanity.'[42] In other words while the allegations about the drugs and crime were in doubt, there was no such equivocation about the link between hemp preparations and madness. All dissenting voices were dismissed and action was insisted upon. The Government of India prohibited the cultivation and use of hemp drugs in Burma and urged other areas of British India to 'discourage the consumption of ganja and bhang by placing restrictions on their cultivation, preparation and retail, and

---

[39] Ibid. 35.   [40] Ibid. 11.   [41] Ibid. 65.   [42] Ibid. 92.

imposing on their use as high a rate of duty as can be levied without inducing illicit practices'.[43]

The reason that the Government of India felt so confident in its assertions about the link between use of cannabis substances and mental illness lies in the statement at the start of this section that 'of the cases of insanity produced by the excessive use of drugs or spirits, by far the largest number must be attributed to the abuse of hemp'. The Government of India felt that it could pronounce on the subject with such clarity and authority because of that number, a clarity and authority that it felt had been established throughout a report that was littered with statistics. Consider the reply from the authorities in the Central Provinces of India.

Dr Beatson, Civil Surgeon Nagpur and superintendent of the asylum reports that out of 317 lunatics received into the asylum since 1864, there were 61 in whom insanity had been occasioned by an immoderate indulgence in ganja. Of these 61, 10 have died, 28 have been discharged cured and 23 remain uncured. He therefore concludes that excess in ganja smoking does produce an insanity which is transient if the habit is relinquished but otherwise permanent.[44]

Similarly, the reply from Mysore quoted the figures of the asylum superintendent Dr Ranking which showed 'that out of a total of 250 admissions in the lunatic asylum in Bangalore during the past five years the use of ganja is assigned as the cause of insanity in 82 cases, but 64 persons of the number so affected subsequently recovered their reason, and were discharged'.[45] The whole report of Dr Penny at the Delhi asylum was included in the reply of the Punjab and a statistical table that traced the percentages of the total treated for hemp related mental disorders in the years 1867–71 was printed. This showed an increasing percentage of those treated to be attributable to cannabis drugs. He also took the trouble to reproduce a reference to the Annual Report of the Lunatic Asylums in Bengal where he had discovered that 'cannabis constitutes 31 per cent of the whole; 78 of the known causes of insanity'.[46]

That these numbers were taken seriously by the central administration is reflected in the fact that all these statistics were reproduced in the summary of the evidence prepared by the Government of India which also included a reproduction of the table of Dr Penny and his observation that 'Of 317 lunatics received into the Nagpur Asylum since 1864, there were 61 in whom insanity had been occasioned by an immoderate use of ganja...

---

[43] 'Papers Relating to the Consumption of Ganja and Other Drugs in India', *British Parliamentary Papers*, vol. 66 (Hansard, London, 1891), 92.

[44] Ibid. 9.　　　　[45] Ibid. 12.　　　　[46] Ibid. 15.

From this result it is inferred that excess in ganja-smoking does produce an insanity which is transient.'[47] The colonial officials in the Government of India, caught in a morass of anecdotes and scare stories on the issue of cannabis, found comfort in the science of the simple statistic. As such it based its conclusions and policy upon these numbers generated by the British doctors in the asylums of India.

These asylums hold the key to understanding why the Government of India gave its official endorsement to the idea that cannabis use resulted in mental illness. Throughout the nineteenth century the British had set up a network of lunatic asylums across colonial India. At first these had been established to separate out Indian soldiers that had gone mad from the rest of the regiment, and later on the British found that they were useful places in which to place those that they found dangerous and disruptive in the local population. As the colonial superintendents at these asylums kept increasingly detailed records of their hospitals and began to collate these into statistical tables in end-of-year reports for their superiors, an alarming conclusion began to emerge. The largest single cause of the mental problems experienced by their patients was cannabis use.[48]

Yet a closer look at the mental hospitals themselves reveals that these apparently solid statistics were in fact no more scientific than the most fabulous of the stories that the Government of India had heard on the subject of cannabis use in the Indian population. The asylums actually created an illusion that there was a problem rather than identified a real issue. There were two stages by which cannabis use and cannabis users became categorized as a social problem in the asylums of colonial India. First, medical officers at the asylums came to believe that cannabis use was linked to insanity in Indians. Second, the officers used the asylum as a site where they could observe cannabis users and establish the distinguishing signs which marked them off as a distinct human type to be watched out for because of their dangerous potential.

The first step in these processes came when the new admission to the hospital was dragged in from the street by the police. The superintendents needed to fill the forms in and chief among the issues on these documents was the 'cause of insanity' section. On the whole the asylums of India filled up with vagrants and the poor and as such there was often great difficulty in getting a hold of accurate data with which to complete this section. Nevertheless the form needed to be completed. Consider the testimony of

[47] Ibid. 88.
[48] For more on the origins of this network see J. Mills, *Madness, Cannabis and Colonialism: The 'Native Only' Lunatic Asylums of British India, 1857 to 1900* (Macmillan, Basingstoke, 2000), 66–128.

Dr Simpson in the asylums report for Bengal in 1874: 'Among the pauper class information as to the cause, unless the case be that of a known ganja-smoker, is often not procurable; and as the formal statement of the cases includes a direct question, an imaginary cause is entered.'[49] He goes on to point out that 'judging from the style of the answers furnished by the police in the descriptive rolls, it would appear that if the man be a ganjah-smoker the drug is invariably put down by them as the cause of insanity'.[50] What he is describing is a process in which the police, who needed to come up with a cause of insanity to complete the forms correctly, often could find no evidence of what had disrupted the behaviour of the individual that they wished to incarcerate. This meant that they would have to make up a cause of insanity, and in such a situation 'ganjah-smoking' was a convenient way of filling the document and one that was likely to be believed.

It was likely to be believed by the British medical officer for all sorts of reasons. The first was that many in India shared the opinion of the Commissioner of Sitapur that preparations of hemp, by virtue of their intoxicating properties, were comparable to alcohol and opium and were therefore an irredeemable evil likely to lead to mental problems.

In his own court Commissioner [*sic*] has seen more than one instance in which the criminal pleaded, in excuse or explanation of violence or murder, that the crime was committed when under the influence of bhang; and there is in his mind no doubt that the use of the drug operates much as intoxicating liquors do in England, by stimulating the passions and weakening the power of self-control.[51]

Then there was the fact that the use of an external stimulant to cause madness suited medical theories of the day that insisted on physiological causes of mental illness. Add to this the fact that the superintendent of the asylum was also likely to be the supervisor of all the other local hospitals and jails, that he was expected to care for all the European patients in the district, that he probably knew little about psychiatry as he was not required to have passed exams in this in order to gain a post in the Indian Medical Service, and the fact that he probably considered all Indians to be a bit mad in the first place and it is easy to see why a simple and quick means of filling in the forms was acceptable to him.

As such the case notes of admission to the lunatic hospitals of India came to read as follows.

---

[49] *Annual Report on the Insane Asylums in Bengal for the Year 1874* (Calcutta, 1875), 16.
[50] Ibid.
[51] 'Papers Relating to the Consumption of Ganja and Other Drugs in India', 48.

Bhugwan Dass. Mania acute. 26. Hindoo. Labour. 23 Feby/ 69.
Certified by Magistrate violent

28 Feb 1869. Probably from bhung. He is very troublesome + destructive. Sent in by City Magistrate of Lucknow.

3rd May. Made over to his friends by order of the committee.[52]

As this is the entire case note it seems that all the information available for Bhugwan Dass is that he was destructive and that this was thought to have been the result of the man's use of a preparation of hemp. The implication of the qualification 'probably' suggests that the medical officer had no direct evidence that hemp was the cause of the man's behaviour yet he was happy to record the conjecture. The case note for Allya Khan reads in a similar way.

Allya Khan. M. Mania. 30. Mussulman. Coolie. 17th Jany/ 63.

1863. Sent in by City Magistrate found wandering about Bazar in City is an inhabitant of Lucknow ... apparently had been smoking and using some drugs to excess was violent on admission.

Discharged much improved. Made over to his friends.

June 10th. Readmitted having thrown himself down a well. Is worse than ever.[53]

Again, there is only a tenuous connection with cannabis preparations yet the case note establishes a link between madness and the use of hemp narcotics.

The first step in establishing at the asylums of India the link between cannabis and mental health problems was that in which superintendents recorded as official verdict the guesses of local informants such as the police. The next step came when the superintendents decided that those individuals in their care were in fact representative of cannabis users as a whole across the country.

Each and all of these forms of Indian hemp act on the nervous system, exercising a peculiar influence over the brain and spinal chord, and their nerves. They also paralyze the sympathetic nervous system, as shown in the arrest of the secretion of the salivary glands ... There is a state of brain produced by over-indulgence in bhang or charas, which corresponds to delirium tremens; sudden suspension of its

[52] Case Book IV, patient no. 38, admitted 23 Feb. 1869. This is a reference to the case notes of the Lucknow Lunatic Asylum (in the private collection of Dr Aditya Kumar of the Agra Mental Hospital). The reference is to the volume containing the case note (the original numbering on the three surviving volumes is IA, II, and IV and this has been retained), to the patient number within that volume, and the date on which that patient was admitted according to the information available on the case note.

[53] Case Book II, patient no. 4, admitted 17 Jan. 1863.

use causing a state of most violent excitement. The patient talks incessantly; pelts those about him with bricks or stones; bites and tears his clothes; and it would be dangerous to approach him...He may die from exhaustion of the brain, or stoppage of the heart's action from paralysis of the sympathetic, or he may gradually recover.[54]

This report is included in the replies of the Bengal government to the inquiry of 1871–2 and is an extract from Dr Penny's report on the Patna asylum. His information is obviously taken from those that he has observed in the hospital. However, he generalizes grandly in his conclusions and talks of 'the brain' or 'the nervous system' rather than specific brains or individual nervous systems. Having universalized his subject he moves on to the effects of hemp and then on to the behaviour of 'the patient' rather than 'a patient', who is violent and dangerous, and indeed liable to sudden death.

This is the crucial step between observing individuals at the asylum and establishing cannabis use and cannabis users as a social problem in general. The individual instance becomes an example of a universal phenomenon, in other words the disordered individual whose odd behaviour has been linked at the asylum with hemp use becomes representative of all hemp users. It did not occur to the doctors that they were in fact viewing a highly unrepresentative sample of cannabis consumers. The ordinary Indian, who enjoyed a smoke or a drink of some hemp preparation while going about his business, never came to the attention of the British. Indeed, it did not occur to the medical officers that they might not be looking at hemp users at all, and that the policemen that they relied upon for data about the origins of an individual's condition might have all sorts of reasons for feeding the British officer information about cannabis. Rather it was the disordered individual available to satisfy the curiosity of the British doctor at the asylum that represented the sole access the colonial administration had to Indians thought to use cannabis. Thus the violence, weakness, and disruption of those in a lunatic asylum came to be regarded as typical of all Indians who used hemp substances.

The next step in the process of creating a social problem out of hemp users came when the asylum doctors began to look for tell-tale signs by which to identify this class of apparently dangerous and volatile people before they could cause any harm. Various accounts show that medical officers used the asylum in colonial India as a window for observing the body of the hemp user and to build up a picture in their own minds of the

[54] 'Papers Relating to the Consumption of Ganja and Other Drugs in India', 14–15.

physical features by which a user could be recognized. Dr Penny, who was mentioned earlier on, took care to set out a description of the physical characteristics of hemp users; 'Old Bhang drinkers, charas and ganja-smokers and majum-eaters are, as a rule, emaciated. They lose vital energy, become impotent, forgetful, weak-minded and melancholy...again charas-smokers are often asthmatic.'[55] Surgeon Hutchinson at Patna recommended looking for 'a peculiar leery look which, when once seen is unmistakable', and pointed out that, 'a confirmed gunjah smoker has frequently dark, purple lips'. Whatever the difficulties of using these indicators he assured the reader that, 'the corn and inhalation will always reveal him'.[56] The asylum was the place where the British medical officer created an image to be attached to a human type or category and it was where the hemp user of the colonial imagination was 'given flesh'.

The final step in this process of creating cannabis use and the cannabis user as social problems is the key one mentioned earlier, the translation of an issue into a statistic. In among the range of data collected at the asylum and compiled in the asylum statistics was information on 'cause of insanity of those admitted'. In Bengal for example, where the statistics collected were most complex, there were 21 possible causes mooted in the various asylums in 1870 and 22 by 1875. They were divided into physical causes and moral causes. Amongst the physical were such factors as 'epilepsy' or 'miscarriage' and among the moral 'grief' or 'family quarrel'. Ganja was always chief among the assigned causes in the known physical causes column in India throughout the 1860s and 1870s.

The passing of comment on the preponderance of hemp narcotics in the statistical table on causes became a routine part of end-of-year statements. For example, the Superintendent of Dullunda commented in 1867 that 'among the causes of admissions, there appear nothing of novelty or special interest. The fact which each succeeding year brings prominently forward, of the prevalence of ganja smoking as a fertile source of insanity is as prominent as ever in the records of 1867.'[57]

In 1871 Surgeon Cutcliffe pointed out in his report on the asylum at Dacca that 'Table no. 4 shows the causes to which the insanity of the patients has been attributed. 33 percent of all the cases are attributed to gunja smoking and 7.18 to spirit drinking.'[58] In 1875 the officer in charge of the asylum in Cuttack pointed out that 'Ganja is reputed as the cause of the majority of the admissions and nearly half of the admissions during the

[55] Ibid. 15.   [56] *Asylums in Bengal for the Year 1868* (Calcutta, 1869), 37.
[57] *Asylums in Bengal for the Year 1867* (Calcutta, 1868), 10.
[58] *Asylums in Bengal for the Year 1870* (Calcutta, 1871), 35.

past ten years into this asylum are attributed to its abuse.'[59] Throughout the 1860s and 1870s it was a routine statistical conclusion in the asylums of colonial India that cannabis preparations were responsible in the majority of cases where the cause of insanity was recorded.

Almost as routine was the casting of doubt on the reliability of such statistical conclusions. In 1871 one superintendent voiced his concern that 'causation is, as usual, very unsatisfactorily noted among the admissions. Antecedent information is commonly difficult to procure. Intemperance is an assigned cause in 9 cases, but with one or two exceptions I doubt whether it can be regarded as in any sense a true cause in this number.'[60] Surgeon Wise admitted in 1872 that

an attempt has been made this year to distinguish between those cases of insanity clearly due to ganjah-smoking and those in which the use of ganjah has only been occasional, and therefore insufficient to excite insanity. The attempt has not been successful. For want of any other reason, it has been necessary to enter under the heading of ganjah several who were merely reported to have indulged in its use.[61]

Dr Simpson, already mentioned for his misgivings about the nature of police information, was content to base an opinion on this information despite his doubts: 'Judging from the style of the answers furnished by the police in the descriptive rolls, it would appear that if the man be a ganjah-smoker the drug is invariably put down by them as the cause of insanity. However this may be, the figures in Table no. 7 impress one with the conviction that ganjah, bhang and alcohol have more to do with the peopling of our asylums than all other cases put together.'[62]

The concern with the accuracy of the statistics was not just restricted to medical officers in Bengal. The superintendent at the Delhi asylum pointed out that, 'I know the difficulties of obtaining information when perhaps the constable who seizes [or] the Thannadar or Deputy Inspector who receives the charge, is himself wanting intelligence.'[63] As late as 1880 Dr Rice at Jubbulpore was still concerned to establish that

the determination of causes of insanity is of considerably greater difficulty than the classification of the variety. Only too often it is impossible to procure any previous history of the patient. Native relatives (even if any exist and are willing to do so)

[59] *Asylums in Bengal for the Year 1875* (Calcutta, 1876), 24.
[60] *Asylums in Bengal for the Year 1871* (Calcutta, 1872), 75.
[61] *Asylums in Bengal for the Year 1872* (Calcutta, 1873), 65.
[62] *Asylums in Bengal for the Year 1874* (Calcutta, 1875), 16.
[63] *Annual Report of the Lunatic Asylums in the Punjab for the Year 1871–72* (Lahore, 1873), 2.

are not skillful in depicting those traits of character previous to his seizure which might tend to show what led to his becoming insane: but too often the man has no known relatives, and 'shots' are made by the neighbours as to the cause of his madness.[64]

It is crucial to note though that despite the constant concern over the relevance and accuracy of the information and of the statistics they were still registered by the non-medical officers reading the reports and policy was generated on the basis of those numbers. In the report for 1873 for example Surgeon-Major Cayley made it clear that 'I fear that not much reliance can be placed on the alleged causes of insanity...it is difficult to ascertain if ganja was the actual cause in so many cases.'[65] However the Judicial Department resolution, written by a civil officer with no medical training upon receipt of the report, ignored the doctor's misgivings about the reliability of the figures. It confidently stated that 'there is little calling for remark on the present report on the types of insanity or its causes. Of the exciting causes of insanity, ganjah-smoking is still shown in the returns for the whole of the Lower Provinces as one of the most frequent; and it is observable that in many cases of re-admission the patients are said to have been confirmed smokers of the drug.' On the basis of this reading of the statistics the Judicial Department's resolution recorded that 'the Lieutenant-Governor is giving special attention to the best means for further augmenting the check (which has been imposed of late years apparently with some success) on the consumption of this most deleterious drug'.[66] In other words the statistics of the asylums were directly responsible for governmental decisions about cannabis use and cannabis users. It did not matter that the medical officers responsible for those statistics actually reported that there were problems with understanding exactly what they signified. Once statistics existed, that which they described existed in the minds of colonial administrators who responded with social policy initiatives.

The government in India came to believe that the lunatic asylum system of the region had generated an authoritative statistic that proved that there was a link between mental illness and cannabis use. It has been suggested here that the numbers produced by the British medical officers at the lunatic asylums had anything but solid or sound foundations. They were in fact based on bad information, administrative expedience, and colonial

[64] *Report on the Lunatic Asylums in the Central Provinces for the Year 1880* (Nagpur, 1881), 7.
[65] *Asylums in Bengal for the Year 1873* (Calcutta, 1874), 63.
[66] Ibid. 3.

misunderstandings of a complex society.[67] Nevertheless, this data came to establish in the minds of many that there was a supposedly scientific and rational basis for asserting that cannabis use led to mental illness. These statistics, and the accusation that they were nothing but falsehoods and fabrications did not, however, simply remain the concern of British administrators in India. By the 1890s they had become the stuff of controversy in the House of Commons in London.

---

[67] For a more detailed version of this argument and its origins see Mills, *Madness, Cannabis and Colonialism*, 43–65. There is a range of studies available that similarly explore the ways that the British in India constructed social categories and social problems. For the criminal tribes see S. Nigam, 'Disciplining and Policing the "Criminals" by Birth, Part I: The Making of a Colonial Stereotype—The Criminal Tribes of North India', *Indian Economic and Social History Review*, 27/2 (1990), and R. Tolen, 'Colonizing and Transforming the Criminal Tribesman: the Salvation Army in British India', in J. Urla and J. Terry (eds.), *Deviant Bodies: Critical Perspectives on Difference in Science and Popular Culture* (Indiana University Press, Bloomington, 1995). Statistics were especially important in the creation of caste categories and are examined in B. Cohn, 'The Census, Social Structure and Objectification in South India' in B. Cohn, *An Anthropologist among the Historians and Other Essays* (Oxford University Press, Oxford, 1987), and A. Appadurai, 'Number in the Colonial Imagination', in C. A. Breckenridge and Peter van der Veer (eds.), *Orientalism and the Postcolonial Predicament: Perspectives on South Asia* (University of Pennsylvania Press, Philadelphia, 1993). This chapter borrows the notions of 'categorization' and 'enumeration' from the latter. The idea that carceral sites were used as observatories for producing information about Indian society as a whole can be found in the context of the prison in D. Arnold, 'The Colonial Prison: Power, Knowledge and Penology in Nineteenth-Century India', in D. Arnold and D. Hardiman (eds.), *Subaltern Studies VIII* (Oxford University Press, 1994).

5

'The lunatic asylums of India are filled with ganja smokers': Ganja in Parliament, 1891–1894

CANNABIS AND THE OPIUM CAMPAIGNERS

Drawing on information from the subcontinent, Mark Stewart MP stood up in the House of Commons on 16 July 1891 'to ask the Under-Secretary of State for India whether his attention has been called to the statement in the *Allahabad Pioneer* of the 10th May last that ganja "which is grown, sold and excised under much the same conditions as opium", is far more harmful than opium, and that "the lunatic asylums of India are filled with ganja smokers" '.[1] He pressed his point, asking further of the Under-Secretary 'whether he is aware that the possession and sale of ganja has been prohibited for many years past in Lower Burma and that the exclusion of the drug was stated in the Excise Report of that province for 1881–2 to have been "of immense benefit to the people" '. The reason for his curiosity was that he wanted to know 'whether he [the Under-Secretary of State] will call the attention of the Government of India to the desirability of extending the same prohibition to the other Provinces of India?'

Sir J. Gorst, the Under-Secretary of State for India, must have known that he was in the midst of a barrage from the anti-opium campaigners. He had already been harangued by another Scottish MP, the representative for Flintshire, about opium use in India and had faced the demand that

---

[1] 'Papers Relating to the Consumption of Ganja and Other Drugs in India', *British Parliamentary Papers*, 66 (Hansard, London, 1891), 3.

'he...ask the Indian Government to withdraw provisions calculated to stimulate the consumption of opium in India, in accordance with the decision of the House of Commons?' He had carefully answered each of the points in that attack and patiently ended with the politician's reassurance that 'it is not the policy of the Government of India to stimulate the consumption of opium or any other intoxicant'. Indeed, Mark Stewart quickly followed up his question on ganja with a request for more information on the fate of 'the Memorial presented to Lord Cross from the Anti-Opium Society on 31st July 1890'. Moreover, government officials looking around the chamber that day might have guessed that temperance issues in the empire were likely to be on their way, as Sir George Campbell of Kirkcaldy was in and about to launch an attack on the Under-Secretary of State for the Colonies on 'the importation of European spirits for the use of natives' into West Africa.

Gorst therefore handled the question on ganja as if it were just another stick with which the temperance and anti-opium campaigners intended to beat him, so he gave little attention to the details of the cannabis question. Yes, he was aware of all that his Right Honourable colleague had pointed out and he would, he offered 'inquire whether the Government of India will propose to take further steps to limit the consumption'. As Gorst had taken the ganja question with a straight bat, Sir J. Kennaway, the member for Honiton in Devon, took up the attack again with an opium googly. 'I beg to ask the First Lord of the Treasury whether his attention has been called to the issue of licences for the sale of opium in Bombay and especially to the provision requiring a certain amount to be sold by the licensee under heavy penalties; whether considering the assurance given that the policy of the Indian Government was to diminish the cultivation and consumption of the drug, he will cause representations to be made to the Government of Bombay so that no such provisions should be inserted in future licenses?'[2]

The history of cannabis and Parliament had begun. But the introduction of the issue into Parliament by a famed and active temperance campaigner in the midst of an ambush on the issue of opium shows that the hemp plant and its preparations were not being considered in their own right, but were instead being lumped together with other narcotics by those that wished to attack all stimulants and narcotics. Mark Stewart was, after all, an experienced temperance campaigner by the 1890s and a member of the vociferous anti-opium campaign that finally cornered the government on the issue in the last decade of the nineteenth century. He had been badgering the

[2] *Hansard's Parliamentary Debates*, 355 (3rd Series), 1395–1412, 16 July 1891.

authorities about opium for almost twenty years and had urged the House of Commons to pass the motion that 'the Imperial policy regulating the opium traffic between India and China should be carefully considered by Her Majesty's Government with a view to gradual withdrawal of the Government of India from the cultivation and manufacture of Opium' as early as 1875.[3] The motion was not passed by the House but this was the first parliamentary move of the anti-opium campaign that was to gather momentum until the 1890s. In 1891 Sir Joseph Pease successfully brought forward the motion in the House of Commons that 'this House is of the opinion that the system by which the Indian opium revenue is raised is morally indefensible, and would urge upon the Indian Government that it should cease to grant licenses for the cultivation of the poppy'.[4] Stewart was still at the forefront of the campaign in this period, speaking alongside Pease for example in the debates on the subject of 3 May 1889 when he took on religious authority and announced that 'the opinion of the Christian Churches in this country is that the Indian Government ought no longer to be the producers and manufacturers of this drug'.[5] This tone had been adopted by Pease, who had argued that 'this trade, demoralizing to so large a portion of mankind, stands in the way of the spread of the Christian faith that we all desire'. In fact, opium was not the only intoxicant to worry Stewart. Since the 1870s he had been a supporter of legislative measures on alcohol, standing for example to speak in support of the Intoxicating Liquors (Scotland) Bill in 1875 and announcing in the following year that in the case of intemperate use of spirits in Ireland 'he would rather that moral suasion were used to remedy the evil complained of but that having failed it was high time to legislate on the subject'.[6]

Indeed, it seems that cannabis was of little real interest to Mark Stewart as an issue in itself and was rather seen as just another intoxicant and just another way of darkening the reputation of the Government of India in the House of Commons by emphasizing its murky dealings in drugs. Stewart had raised the subject of ganja only once before in begging 'to ask the Under-Secretary of State if he can inform the House of the number of shops or houses in each province of British India licensed for the retail sale of opium, ganja, and bhang respectively and in how many of these opium

[3] Ibid., 225 (3rd Series), 571, 25 June 1875.
[4] J. Rowntree, *The Opium Habit in the East: a study of the evidence given to the Royal Commission on Opium 1893/4* (King, London, 1895), 4.
[5] *Hansard*, 335 (3rd Series), 1174, 3 May 1889.
[6] Ibid., 230 (3rd Series), 1351, 12 July 1876.

is allowed to be smoked or otherwise consumed on the premises'.[7] Again, the focus of this query seems to have been on opium even though cannabis products were briefly mentioned. Indeed, he never bothered with the subject of cannabis preparations again after his question about the lunatic asylums of India in 1891 although he did continue to concentrate on the issue of opium, even at one point confronting Gladstone on the subject and demanding to know 'if it is the intention of Her Majesty's Government to bring in a Bill, with a view to legislation, on the opium question this Session, in accordance with the Resolution passed by this House in 1891?'[8]

It was one of Stewart's colleagues in Parliament, William Sproston Caine, who instead took up the issue of cannabis use in India. On the face of it, Caine and Stewart were unlikely colleagues. The latter was a member of the old world as he was from Scottish aristocracy as a member of the Stewart clan of Kircudbrightshire in the lowland borders. The former on the other hand was very much new money and a product of the Victorian world as his family had made its fortune in iron ore mining in Cheshire. What they did have in common were questionable electoral histories and a commitment to temperance campaigning. Stewart, for all his moral purpose on the issues of intoxication, was a rather more controversial figure when it came to democratic practices. Declared the winner of the Wigtown Burroughs seat in 1874, he had to face the embarrassment of a parliamentary investigation of the election and indeed the humiliation of its conclusion that eight of Stewart's votes were not admissible. As he had only won by two votes, he lost the seat. However, George Young, the successful candidate was soon promoted to be a judge of the Court of Session and in the resulting by-election Stewart won by a majority of eight votes. Again the election was scrutinized. His majority was reduced to two votes.[9] In 1880 he defeated John McLaren but the election was declared void and neither candidate stood for re-election.[10] Stewart re-entered Parliament in 1885 for Kircudbrightshire and held it until 1906 when he was dumped by the electorate. He made his last appearance in 1910 when he was re-elected in January but on this occasion he chose not to see out his term of office as he retired at the end of the year.[11] Caine, while not suffering the indignities of scrutinized election results that dogged the early parliamentary career of Stewart, did suffer repeated rejection by the electors. He unsuccessfully

[7] Ibid., 342 (3rd Series), 713, 13 Mar. 1890.
[8] Ibid., 9 (4th Series), 1454, 9 Mar. 1893.
[9] F. Craig, *British Electoral Facts 1832–1987* (Gower, Aldershot, 1989), 206.
[10] F. Craig, *British Parliamentary Election Results 1832–1885* (Dartmouth, Aldershot, 1989), 564.
[11] M. Stenton and S. Lees, *Who's Who of British Members of Parliament*, vol. ii (Harvester, Brighton, 1978), 237.

contested Liverpool both in 1873 and 1874 and failed to secure Tottenham in 1885. He was elected in Scarborough and served there between 1880 and 1885, and also acted as MP for Barrow in Furness between 1886 and 1890 when he failed to gain re-election. He won a seat at Bradford in 1892 but lost it in 1895 but did make his way back for a final hurrah and sat as MP for Camborne from 1900 until his death in 1903. When in Parliament however, he did gain recognition and served as Civil Lord of the Admiralty in 1884–5 and as Liberal Unionist Chief Whip from 1886 to 1890.

While Caine and Stewart are unlikely to have spent much time chatting about the shadows in their political careers, they did have the other common interest of temperance reform. Caine was brought up as a Baptist and he came to serve as president of such institutions as the Baptist Total Abstinence Society and the National Temperance Federation. His commitment to issues of temperance was such that at one point he resigned his seat in the House over the matter of compensation for public-house licence holders and he was appointed to the Royal Commission on liquor licensing laws that sat between 1896 and 1899. Significantly, he visited India and in total travelled there three times in his life and he found plenty of time to stick his nose into questions relating to temperance in that country. His biography claims that while in Bombay on his first visit he was approached by 'a large number of educated Hindoos who called his attention to the abuses of the Excise Administration'.[12] He had visited the conference of the Indian National Congress in Allahabad in 1888 as an advocate of more self-rule for India and it is likely that he made his temperance interests known to Indians then. They had approached the right man as Caine was unable to resist the opportunity to criticize the Government of India's policies on intoxicants. When back in Britain and in parliament he planned an attack together with his fellow temperance MP Samuel Smith and they formed the Anglo-Indian Temperance Association of which Caine took the post of Honorary Secretary, a position he held until the end of his life. On 30 April 1889 they offered the following resolution which was put to the ballot in the House of Commons.

In opinion of this House, the fiscal system of the GOI leads to the establishment of spirit distilleries, liquor, and opium shops in large numbers of places, where, till recently, they never existed, in defiance of native opinion and the protests of inhabitants and that such increased facilities for drinking produce a steadily increased consumption, and spread misery and ruin among the industrial classes of India

[12] J. Newton, *WS Caine MP: A Biography* (Nisbet, London, 1907), 236.

calling for immediate action on the part of the GOI with a view to their abate-ment.[13]

The resolution was carried, and the result was the Government of India was contacted and asked to defend its position by the Secretary of State for India, which it did in 1890 through an attack on the alleged misrepresentations that Caine had relied upon.

Indeed, Caine's experiences in India had not simply allowed him to investigate the issues of spirits and opium as he seems to have formed an opinion on all of the intoxicants used in the country. He was no simple across-the-board killjoy and his biographer speaks of his approval of one beverage: 'Mr Caine frequently denounced the mistaken policy of taxing the toddy-palm. The toddy-palm yields a liquid which for ages has formed one of the staple articles of food of the poorer classes in India. Whilst fresh it is perfectly innocuous and wholesome. When fermentation takes place, the result is only a slightly intoxicating beverage.'[14] There was no such treatment for cannabis, which Caine denounced as 'the most horrible intoxicant the world has yet produced'.[15] Even when cashing in on his Indian experiences by writing a guidebook for travellers to South Asia he still found the time to rail against intoxicants. While describing things to do on a wander around Lucknow he inserted the following passage.

Here and there throughout the bazar are little shops whose entire stock consists of a small lump of greenish pudding, which is being retailed out in tiny cubes. This is another 'Government monopoly' and is majoon, a preparation of the deadly bhang or Indian hemp known in Turkey and Egypt as Haseesh, the most horrible intoxicant the world has yet produced. In Egypt, its importation and sale is absolutely forbidden and a costly preventive service is maintained to suppress smuggling of it by Greek adventurers; but a Christian Government is wiser in its generation and gets a comfortable income out of its sale. When an Indian wants to commit some horrible crime, such as murder or wife mutilation, he prepares himself for it with two anna's worth of bhang from a government majoon shop. The little rooms, open to the street, of which the sole furniture is some matting and a few Hukas, are churras or Chandu shops, farmed out by the government of India to provide another form of Indian hemp intoxication which is smoked instead of eaten.

This description was of course closely followed by an account of drinking dens and opium parlours. Fast on the description of cannabis users, he

---

[13] J. Newton, *WS Caine MP: A Biography* (Nisbet, London, 1907), 237.

[14] Ibid. 241.

[15] W. S. Caine, *Picturesque India: A Handbook for European Travellers* (Routledge, London, 1890), 292.

creates the image of 'the groups of noisy men seated on the floor [who] are drinking ardent spirits of the worst description, absolutely forbidden to the British soldier, but sold retail to natives at three farthings a gill, of which two farthings go to the exchequer' who were sat nearby the 'large native house . . . through a door of which streams in and out a swarm of customers. It is perhaps three o'clock in the afternoon. Entering with them, you will find yourself in a spacious but very dirty courtyard, round which are ranged fifteen or twenty small rooms. The stench is sickening, the swarm of flies intolerable, and there is something strange and weird in the faces of those coming in from the street. This is the establishment of another Government contractor, the opium farmer.' Cannabis, for Caine, was tied together with his fears about alcohol and opium in India and was caught up in his political opposition to the colonial government there.

THE OPIUM COMMISSION AND THE INDIAN HEMP DRUGS COMMISSION OF 1893/4

On his return from India and his election at Bradford in 1892 Caine settled back into catching up with parliamentary life. The Government of India had promised a response to Mark Stewart's question in 1891 so Caine stood up in the Commons on 14 February 1893 in order to 'beg to ask the Under-Secretary of State for India whether the Indian Government has yet forwarded to the India Office the further Despatch dealing with the case of ganja and other drugs, promised in paragraph 4 of its Despatch, dated 14th October 1891?' He evidently suspected the Government of India of dragging its feet but instead learnt from George Russell, who was now the Under-Secretary of State for India, that it had indeed arrived accompanied by a range of papers and that it would be 'laid upon the Table if my hon. Friend will move for them'.[16] Caine did indeed apply to see the report and it was sent for printing on 8 March.

Once back in the Commons, Caine quickly joined in with the anti-opium campaign, in fact just a couple of days before the ganja report was sent for printing he had risen in the House of Commons to badger the government about opium smoking dens in the North-West Provinces of India.[17] Indeed, Caine had been in regular correspondence with the campaigners while he was in India and Sir Joseph Pease had quoted a letter

[16] *Hansard*, 8 (4th Series), 1360, 14 Feb. 1893.
[17] Ibid., 9 (4th Series), 1087, 6 Mar. 1893.

from him while attacking the government on the issue of opium with the support of Mark Stewart back in May 1889. In this letter Caine had insisted that 'I have been in East-end gin palaces on Saturday nights, I have seen men in various stages of delirium tremens, I have visited many idiot and lunatic asylums but I have never seen such horrible destruction of God's image in the face of man as I saw in the Government opium dens of Lucknow.'[18]

With his experience of attacking the government on alcohol and opium issues in India, and with a personal belief in the evils of cannabis based on his experiences in South Asia, it is little surprise that it was Caine that took up the issue that Stewart had identified but quickly dropped. Before even seeing the response to Mark Stewart's question from the Government of India he piped up again, this time to demand action. 'I beg to ask the Under-Secretary of State for India if the Secretary of State for India will instruct the Government of India to create a Commission of Experts to inquire into, and report upon, the cultivation of and trade in all preparations of hemp drugs in Bengal, the effect of their consumption upon the social and moral condition of the people, and the desirability of prohibiting its growth and sale.' He also insisted that 'the Commission shall be partly composed of non-official natives of India'.[19] To what seems to have been his surprise, George Russell stood up and declared 'the Secretary of State proposes to request the Viceroy to appoint a Commission to inquire into the cultivation and trade in hemp drugs and he will be glad if the result of their inquiry is to show that further restrictions can be placed upon the sale and consumption of these drugs'. The Indian Hemp Drugs Commission (IHDC) had been established, although Caine seems not to have expected this as he had a resolution on the subject lined up on the Order Book that he had to arrange to be withdrawn.[20] J. Gorst, who had been the Under-Secretary of State for India back in 1891, spotted that this was sudden and unexpected given the far greater interest of the House in other drugs, so he

[18] *Hansard*, 335 (3rd Series), 1160, 3 May 1889.

[19] Ibid., 9 (4th Series), 822, 2 Mar. 1893.

[20] This motion moved that 'In the opinion of this House the growth, cultivation and sale of bhang, ganja, charas and other preparations of hemp by the Provincial Governments of India produce much misery, poverty, insanity and moral deterioration among the people of India; and whereas similar results in Turkey, Egypt and Greece have led to the absolute prohibition in those countries of the manufacture and common sale of hemp drugs, it is desirable that the Secretary of State for India should order a commission of experts to enquire into and report upon the cultivation of and trade in all preparations of hemp drugs in Bengal, the effect of their consumption upon the people of that presidency and the desirability of the prohibition of their sale; not less than one half of such commission to be composed of non-official natives of India', *Abkari* 14 (July 1893), 111.

asked, 'will the question of opium be considered by the Commission?' The answer was in the negative and it was not until June of that year that the government authorized a royal commission on opium.[21] Caine's questions and attention to the subject meant that the House of Commons had secured an investigation into cannabis products before MPs managed to get one into opium. He was dogged in ensuring that the matter was seen to as a matter of urgency as well, asking questions throughout June about who was going to be on the Commission and finally receiving his answer on 7 July. But the suspicion lingers that both for Stewart and for Caine, and indeed for the government, the cannabis issue was simply caught up in the politics of opium.

This was an important year in Parliament. Gladstone presented it with the Home Rule Bill, and controversy ensued as the Commons approved it twice and the Lords rejected it once. The opium issue was also coming to a head in this year. The Society for the Suppression of the Opium Trade, under a new secretary, J. G. Alexander, organized a series of public meetings and petitions from 1889 onwards and in total over 200,000 signatures were collected.[22] One of the most important of those gathered by opponents of the drug was of 5,000 British doctors that asserted that 'the habit of opium smoking or of opium eating is morally and physically debasing'.[23] It was thought that even key members of the government, such as the Foreign Secretary Edward Grey and George Russell, the Parliamentary Secretary for India, were supporters of the anti-opium movement. The parliamentary agitators let it be known that a motion was to appear. When Alfred Webb duly introduced the motion, supported by the veteran Sir Joseph Pease, it suggested that the Government of India take steps to end the production and export of opium immediately and that a royal commission be established. This commission would investigate how the cost to the Indian economy of the end of the trade could be made good by reforms in the administration of India, by a new set of economic policies, and even by a grant from the British Exchequer. In other words, the motion was not simply directed at the opium trade but at the system of government in India as well. If passed and made effective the motion would not simply cost money in terms of lost opium revenue, but it would mean additional

---

[21] Rowntree, *Opium Habit in the East*, 4.

[22] D. Owen, *British Opium Policy in China and India* (Archon, New Haven, 1968), 314. For other details of activities of the anti-opium campaigners see V. Berridge and G. Edwards, *Opium and the People: Opiate Use in Nineteenth Century England* (Allen Lane, London, 1981), 173–205; M. Booth, *Opium: a history* (Simon & Schuster, London, 1996), 155–7.

[23] *Hansard*, 14 (4th Series), 595, 30 June 1893.

expenditure to ensure that with the ending of the trade 'the people of India ought not to be called upon to bear the cost involved'.[24]

The opium trade was an integral feature of the finances of Britain's Asian empire. The administration of India was a costly and secretive affair, apparently under the scrutiny of Parliament but in fact introduced there only annually and in the summer, a time when MPs usually found more pleasant tasks to attend to. Indeed this was something that the opium campaigners complained of: 'this House at the present moment has no more control over the Indian finances than the man in the street. The Indian Debate comes on generally in the month of August and hardly any of us have found much more than a quorum of the House sitting when the whole of this vast system of finance has to be looked at.'[25] The government therefore had no intention of giving up the trade or indeed of suddenly subjecting the financial system of India to the sustained scrutiny of the House of Commons. However, it needed to find responses to the growing pressure and to take the steam out of the movement in parliament.

Gladstone therefore offered an alternative motion in which a royal commission was granted, but on the government's terms. No mention was made of India's financial systems. The question for the Commission was not of what to do once the opium trade was abolished but whether the trade might be abolished at all and what the impact of this abolition would be on the Indian economy. The Commission was also to investigate 'the consumption of opium by the different races and in the different districts of India and the effect of such consumption on the moral and physical condition of the people'.[26] This was not what the committed campaigners wanted at all, as opium was far less of a problem in India than in China, where addiction was thought to be rife and to which the Government of India supplied the bulk of its opium output in contravention of Chinese law. They therefore voted against Gladstone but many in the House felt that the government had been seen to act and approved Gladstone's rather than Webb's motion by 184 votes to 105. Joshua Rowntree, writing for the Society for the Suppression of the Opium Trade, noted that the Royal Commission had been 'diverted from the larger issue at stake to a minor one'.[27]

With diversionary tactics as the name of the government's game on the opium question and with a policy of dissipating interest in the major issues by presenting other distractions it is easy to see why cannabis so suddenly

[24] *Hansard*, 14 (4th Series), 591, 30 June 1893.
[25] Sir Joseph Pease, ibid., 612.
[26] W. E. Gladstone ibid., 626.
[27] Rowntree, *Opium Habit in the East*, 5.

merited an inquiry all of its own. Providing this investigation when it did, the government gave an appearance of activity on drugs issues in the run-up to the debate about the opium motion in Parliament. The cannabis inquiry also acted to occupy and to mollify William Caine. As a campaigner that could claim direct experience of the situation in India, he was an important contributor to the parliamentary attacks, and indeed had asked probing questions of the government early in 1893 about the consumption of opium in South Asia and about dens of users in Bombay. However, with the issue of the Cannabis Commission to divert his attention he took no part in the opium motion debates. In fact his only contribution to the argument in Parliament was some way short of significant as he stood one week after the main debate to ask whether arrangements for establishing the Opium Commission were being made 'by telegraph or letter?'[28] Indeed, this was not his first question that day, as he had already enquired after the composition of the Bengal Ganja Commission, a query that he had already made three times in the previous month, a month when the House was raging but he was silent about opium.

Indeed, the suspicion that the IHDC was a diversionary tactic on the part of the Government of India and the British government remains when the actions of key officials in India are considered in the early 1890s. It appears that senior officials were themselves stirring up a fuss over cannabis. Sir William Hunter for example was reported in the Indian press in 1892 as declaring that 'one result of a prohibition of the opium traffic in India would be to drive the people who consumed that drug to the use of one much more pernicious'.[29] The feared replacement for opium was of course cannabis. There was also a passing reference in the *Indian Mirror* to the idea that the Lieutenant-Governor of Bengal himself was behind the IHDC as it reported that '*The Englishman* was in duty bound to say recently that the Hemp Commission appointed by the House of Commons, was due to a proposal of Sir Charles Elliott submitted to the Government of India'.[30] If this had been the case then it would have marked a very interesting turn-around in Elliott's approach to cannabis as it had been noted in the official Resolution on the Excise Report of 1890–1 that 'the Lieutenant-Governor must decline to endorse Mr Westmacott's sweeping condemnation of ganja as a most pernicious article. Sir Charles Elliott has known many instances of its steady and regular use by most respectable people who find themselves

---

[28] *Hansard*, 14 (4th Series), 1057, 7 July 1893.

[29] *Times of India* quoted in *Abkari: The Quarterly Organ of the Anglo-Indian Temperance Association*, 11 (1892), 181.

[30] *Indian Mirror* quoted in *Abkari*, 14 (1893), 129.

able to do hard work with its help and who feel no injurious effects from it.'[31] The suggestion that Elliott had been quietly arranging for the IHDC would make William Caine a dupe of the Government of India's machinations. If such a commission had already been discussed or even arranged by the GOI then this would explain how the Secretary of State for India could offer it so suddenly and in a manner so apparently out of the blue that even Caine seemed surprised by its announcement. It would also fit in with the policy of obfuscation on the issue of drugs pursued by the British government and the Government of India whose revenues were under threat.

Of course there were many in India that did believe that cannabis was an evil on a par with or even superior to opium and Chapter 4 showed that there were often strong convictions on the subject amongst the British in India. However, the reasons why the Government of India might have found it expedient to focus attention on cannabis are readily apparent. The two possible reasons for this policy would have been first, as already mentioned, a desire to complicate the opium issue by introducing another set of substances into the debate. A second objective in attracting attention to the issue of hemp drugs was to offer them as a sacrifice to temperance campaigners that would not have such a serious impact on excise revenue as would prohibition of opium. Cannabis was a significant source of income, especially in Bengal where it accounted for about a fifth of the revenue from internal customs. But the income from this was nothing compared to that from the exports of opium that were the target of the campaigners who objected to the financing of the empire in Asia by the sale of drugs from India to China. Indeed, this possibility that cannabis was being used as a diversion or indeed even being offered up as a sacrifice was discussed at the time in an article that worried about the possibility that 'ganja is made to do duty as a stalking-horse'.

Some people who have sailed along very comfortably for a good many years without troubling themselves about the vices of the people have suddenly discovered what a very dreadful thing ganja-smoking is and how hideously wrong the anti-opium party are for not attacking this evil instead of the other…the suggestion that they should leave off fighting the opium evil to attack ganja is too absurd to be listened to for a moment. As well try to divert the attention of a man who is killing a cobra to a nest of scorpions close by, as to divert the energies of the anti-opium party at this crisis to the local evil of ganja-smoking.[32]

[31] *Indian Mirror* quoted in *Abkari*, 14 (1893), 129.
[32] *Banner of Asia* quoted in *Abkari*, 11 (1892), 181–2.

The IHDC also acted to attract attention in India away from the Royal Commission on Opium. The latter was conducted in India between November 1893 and February 1894 while the Cannabis Commission held its meetings in the country between 22 August and 6 October 1893 and also between 25 October 1893 and 25 April 1894. In other words the Cannabis Commission both anticipated the Opium Commission and accompanied it. The Opium Commission had as a leading member Sir James Lyall, the former Lieutenant-Governor of the Punjab, while the cannabis inquiry was headed by the First Financial Commissioner of the same region. The Cannabis Commission interviewed 1,193 witnesses in conjunction with its inquiries and collected eight volumes of evidence. The Opium Commission asked questions of 723 people and produced seven volumes. Much the same questions were asked about opium as were of cannabis and for most of the time the questions were asked of the same people. Cannabis and opium had become jumbled together in the minds of the campaigners while agitating for investigations and were deliberately linked by the Government of India in their strategies of complicating and confusing the issue of India and drugs revenues.

THE INDIAN HEMP DRUGS COMMISSION (IHDC)

Whatever the origins of the Indian Hemp Drugs Commission, its members seem to have taken the job seriously enough. The Indian members of the Commission, all of whom were 'non-official' as a result of William Caine's stipulation, were, however, unlikely to want to cause too much of a stir. Raja Soshi Sikhareswar Roy was a landowner, a zamindar, in Rajshahi which was one of the hemp growing districts of East Bengal and indeed was noted for his commitment to 'the improvement of agricultural methods in the province'.[33] The British had granted him the title Raja in 1889 and would go on to promote him to the status of Raja Bahadur in 1896. Lal Chand was a prominent lawyer in the Punjab where he was an Advocate of the Chief Court and a Fellow of the University. He was given the title Rai Bahadur by the British in 1904.[34] Perhaps most grand of the three 'non-official' gentlemen was Kanwar Harnam Singh. The youngest son of His Highness Raja-i-Rajgan of Kapurthala, he had proved himself an able agricultural manager and had run the family's estates in Oudh for almost

---

[33] *Who's Who in India 1911* (Newul Kishore, Lucknow, 1911), part v, p. 3.
[34] Ibid., part iii, p. 126.

twenty years. He was made a CIE in 1885 and a KCIE in 1899 and was granted the title Raja in 1907. A Christian convert, his sons all served the British Empire, one as a colonial officer in the Punjab, one as a bureaucrat in the Imperial Education Department, and a third as a doctor in the Indian Medical Service.[35] The Indians may not have been 'officials' in the Government of India but their loyalty to it was amply rewarded in their lifetimes and their interests and those of their families remained closely tied to it.

The official members of the inquiry were all successful, British career officers in the Government of India. The President of the Commission was Mackworth Young, the First Financial Commissioner of the Punjab, and the Secretary was H. J. McIntosh, who was an Under-Secretary in the Financial and Municipal Department of Bengal. H. T. Ommanney was a District Collector in the Bombay Presidency and A. H. L. Fraser was a District Commissioner in the Central Provinces. The medical presence on the Commission was Surgeon-Major Warden, who was one of William O'Shaughnessy's successors as Professor of Chemistry in Calcutta and as Chemical Examiner to the Government of Bengal.

The scope for these men was clearly defined. They had to establish the extent to which both wild and cultivated hemp was grown, they had to define the different drugs made from the crops, and they needed to report on who was using these substances. They were told to find out exactly what the physical effects of the different preparations were and the Commission was specifically pointed towards the issue of insanity arising from use of cannabis drugs. But they were also reminded to bear in mind that the drugs might also be harmless. Finally, they had to establish the system of taxing the trade of the drugs in each part of India and to show how the various administrations in India raised revenue from the trade. They were told to come up with recommendations, but if they chose to prohibit cannabis intoxicants they had to report on the possibility of social and political unrest as a result of this and also on the alternative intoxicants that those deprived of their dose of hemp drugs might turn to.

The Commission was most thorough and compiled eight volumes of witness statements and conclusions in the seven months of its life. On the first tour, the Commission arrived at Allahabad on 22 August 1893, Jubbulpore on 2 September, Poona on 12 September, and on to Madras for 22 September, taking in a meeting with the Resident at Mysore in Bangalore on the way. In other words, in the weather of the monsoon months they had

[35] *Who's Who in India 1911* (Newul Kishore, Lucknow, 1911), part iii, p. 65.

travelled a considerable part of the way down and across India. They split up when they finished in Madras, with the two groups heading back across the country to Bombay via different routes. They met up a week after leaving Madras and then took a week to head all the way back to Simla in the Himalayas, taking in the mountains of Rajasthan from Mount Abu and Delhi on the way. A second tour, this time devoted to interviews with witnesses, kicked off on 25 October and continued until 18 April.

Indeed, the work at times seemed to threaten the health of some of the Commissioners. Raja Soshi Sikhareswar managed only 44 of the 83 days of the first tour while Lala Nihal Chand managed a slightly better 49. Kanwar Harnam Singh did all of them but seemed to suffer for it as he then took on only 78 of the 183 days of the second tour. Raja Soshi Sikhareswar Roy fared better but only did 112 days of the stint, while Lala Nihal Chand seemed entirely exhausted by illness at this point and in fact attended interviews for only a fortnight in November and a week in April. The other officers all seem to have gamely soldiered through full helpings of both tours, clocking up 266 days of Commission each. All Commissioners had, however, regained their health in time for the writing up of the report in Simla in May of 1894.

Many stories emerged on the tours that emphasized just how diverse was the picture of cannabis use in India. In Bombay for example, the Collector of Land Revenue and Customs wrote a lengthy report in which he regaled the Commission with details of exactly how embedded cannabis preparations were in Indian culture. 'The properties of the bhang plant, its power to suppress the appetites, its virtues as a febrifuge, and its thought-bracing qualities show that the bhang leaf is the home of the great Yogi or brooding ascetic Mahadev,' claimed Campbell, who asserted that 'such holiness and such evil-scaring powers must give bhang a high place among lucky objects'. Preparations of cannabis were central to Hindu legend: 'Shiva on fire with the poison churned from the ocean was cooled by bhang. At another time, enraged by family worries, the god withdrew to the fields. The cool shade of a plant soothed him. He crushed and ate of the leaves, and the bhang refreshed him. For these two benefits bhang is shankarpriya, the beloved of Mahadev.'

Because of these religious properties the drugs were used as a part of all manner of rituals and celebrations. Marriages were sealed with the use of cannabis preparations:

So evil scaring and therefore luck bringing a plant must play an important part in the rites required to clear away evil influences. During the great spirit time of marriage in Bombay among almost all of the higher classes of Gujarat Hindus, of the Jain as well as of the Brahmanic sects, the supplies sent by the family of the bride to the bridegroom's party during their seven days' sojourn includes a supply of bhang. The name of the father who neglects to send bhang is held in contempt. Again, after the wedding when the bridegroom and his friends are entertained at the house of the bride, richly spiced bhang is drunk by the guests. The Gujarat Mussalman bride before and after marriage drinks a preparation of bhang.

Campbell also mentioned that oaths were taken with the hand on the cannabis leaf and that during eclipses, war, and times when the rains failed bhang was offered to the gods. Indeed, the drugs were not just part of Hindu culture and he was concerned to show that Muslims in the west of India also approved of bhang: 'to the follower of the later religion of Islam the holy spirit in bhang is not the spirit of the Almighty. It is the spirit of the great prophet Khizr or Elijah.' Both Muslims and Hindus believed, asserted Campbell, that cannabis preparations dulled the pangs of hunger, helped to cure madness, calmed panic, gave comfort in times of trouble and indeed allowed even the most humble to experience heaven. He ended his note by quoting a local saying, 'we drank bhang and the mystery I am, He grew plain. So grand a result, so tiny a sin.'[36]

Indeed, cannabis preparations were not simply part of ancient rituals but had become caught up in the religious revivalism of the latter part of the nineteenth century. One document in the IHDC collection detailed Trinath worship in Eastern Bengal. Started in 1867 by a former policeman, Ananda Chandra Kali, the focus of the worship was the Hindu holy trinity Brahma, Vishnu, and Shiva ('Tri' means three and 'Nath' means lord in Sanskrit). Crucially, however, the rituals were intended to socially unite the divided Hindu community by appealing to the rich and poor and to all of the various local sects and castes. Ananda Chandra therefore wanted to keep his ceremony simple and cheap so he focused on the consumption of three articles that all could afford from the local market: oil, betel leaf, and ganja.

The votaries should assemble at night and worship with flowers. The ganja should be washed in the manner in which people wash ganja for smoking. The worshipper must fill three chillums with equal quantities of ganja, observing due awe and reverence. When all the worshippers are assembled the lamp should be lit with three wicks and the praises of Trinath should be sung. As long as the wicks

---

[36] 'Note by Mr J. M. Campbell, Collector of Land Revenue and Customs and Opium, Bombay, on the Religion of Hemp', in *Report of the Indian Hemp Drugs Commission 1893–4* (Simla, 1894), iii. 250–2.

burn, the god should be worshipped and his praises chanted. The god should be reverentially bowed to at the close of the ouja. When the reading of the Panchali is finished, those that will not show respect to the Prasad (the offering which has been accepted by the god) i.e. chillum of ganja, shall be consigned to eternal hell, and the sincere worshippers shall go to heaven.

The Inspector of Excise who wrote this report, Abhilas Chandra Mukerji, explained that the worship had quickly spread because it appealed to the many ganja smokers of the region as it legitimized their habit. Indeed, he speculated that Ananda Chandra, the high priest of the Trinath rituals, had just such an agenda in mind when he first set up his temple: 'being a ganja-smoker himself, Ananda Kali may have also thought that by introducing the worship he would be able to save the ganja-smokers from disrepute, as then ganja could be consumed in the name of a god and under colour of doing a religious or pious act'. Whatever the motives behind the form of the religion it certainly seems to have caught on and the Inspector mentions ten districts in eastern Bengal where it was popular. It comes as no surprise to find that many of these districts, such as Bogra, Backergunge, and Noakhali were mentioned by Hem Chunder Kerr back in the 1870s as being key ganja producing regions.[37]

However, while the IHDC report does contain plenty of evidence that cannabis preparations were a welcome and integral part of Indian culture it also shows that elements in various communities rejected them. The Commission member, Lala Nihal Chand, collected together a number of songs and sayings from among the volumes of evidence. In the North-West Provinces for example there was a saying that 'if one smokes charas, one's learning is diminished, the seed is burnt up within, coughing goes on till one's belly bursts, and one's face grows red like that of a monkey'. In the Punjab, it was not redness of face that was the problem but quite the opposite: 'Whoever smokes ganja, his face grows pale, | His wife will complain he is impotent, | His brother will say he is afflicted with pain, | But the smoker will turn to his chillum again.' Of the rhyming warnings, the best comes from Sind.

> It is not charas but a curse
> It burns the chest and heart to its worse.
> It brings on dimness of the eyes
> To phlegm and cough it must give rise.
> To blind the eyes it never fails

[37] 'Note by Babu Abhilas Chandra Mukerji, Second Inspector of Excise, on the Origin and History of Trinath Worship in Eastern Bengal', ibid., iii. 253–4.

Or cripple limbs that once were hale.
In what but death, ends its sad tale?[38]

While the IHDC sparked off these cultural observations, it also gathered evidence on the social and economic concerns that had emerged during the century. The stories of smuggling and of tax evasion surfaced again. Some of the most urgent reports came from Burma, which was administered from British India during this period. The British had made possession of the drug in Burma illegal in the 1870s but this had not stopped Indians working in the region from wanting cannabis. As R. G. Culloden, the Superintendent of the Preventive Service in Rangoon explained, 'that there exists a demand for the article and that high prices are paid for it no one can deny; this is testified to by the many attempts that are made to smuggle it into the country, and on which even the heavy penalties inflicted on detected cases do not appear to have any deterrent effect'. He cited a number of stories to show how corrupting the illegal demand for cannabis substances could be.

On the 21st August last as much as 11760 tolas of ganja were found in two cases landed as passengers luggage ex SS Nowshera from Madras. The gunner of Brooking Street wharf was implicated as on landing those boxes he declared that they belonged to him. He was sentenced by the Magistrate to three months' imprisonment and to pay a fine of Rs. 500. His accomplice, a native, who brought the ganja by the steamer as his luggage was awarded two months' imprisonment.

Indeed, one of the problems of controlling the illegal trade was that the police and army were among the largest consumers of the drug. Culloden noticed that 'the attempts at smuggling have been more frequent since the introduction of the Punjabi element in the police force; this is no doubt owing to a greater demand for the article' and he recalled one instance of an arrest in the military:

A Madrassi sepoy was once brought up for being in possession of 3 tolas weight of ganja, he cried as though his very existence was at stake when told that the drug would be confiscated. He said that if it was taken from him, he would be unable to perform his duties and as he was ordered to a station in Upper Burma where it was impossible to obtain it he would die.[39]

Elsewhere in India rumours circulated of the illegal trade in the drugs. In the Central Provinces the Deputy Commissioner of Bhandara reported

[38] 'Note of Dissent by Lala Nihal Chand', ibid., i. 401–2.
[39] 'Memorandum by Mr R. G. Culloden, Assistant Collector of Customs and Superintendent of the Preventive Service Rangoon, on the Smuggling of Ganja into Rangoon', ibid., iii. 255–6.

that 'it is said that in the zemindaries [estates] on the south-eastern border of the district there used to be a good deal of ganja cultivation which has now been stopped and that this ganja used formerly to be introduced into this district'.[40] In Sind the British officers blamed the local princely state for the illicit trade in their region: 'a certain limited amount of smuggling of bhang takes place from Khairpur state, which is adjacent to the Hyderabad, Shikarpur and Thar and Parkar districts, and the reason for this is that the hemp plant is cultivated and bhang manufactured and sold without any restriction in Khairpur'.[41] In Bengal, the Commissioner of Excise complained that 'various attempts have from time to time been made to stop smuggling from the Garhjat and with varying success... in 1878 cultivation of ganja was prohibited within three miles of the frontier, and this was followed by a considerable increase in the consumption of the Rajshahi drug in all the three districts'. He also had the headache of a large market for the drug from Garhjat to contend with, however.

The drug is in great demand with the priests of the famous shrine of Juggernath, and is affected by the attendants of other Orissa temples. It is usually brought in small quantities by pilgrims, mendicants, and others as an acceptable offering to the priests. The offence is most rife in Puri.[42]

Indeed, the issue of crime came up in other forms familiar from the report of 1872 and the IHDC again considered the question of 'the unpremeditated crimes of violence to which intoxication may give rise'.[43] There were plenty who reasoned that it was possible. Mr Knyvett, the District Superintendent of Police in Saharanpur, for example declared that 'the excessive indulgence in either of these three drugs by a person who is not an habitual criminal is liable to incite to unpremeditated crime'[44] and Mr Tucker of the police at Dinajpur was equally convinced that 'excessive indulgence in ganja incites a man to unpremeditated crime, the effects of rashness and violence of temper caused by smoking it'.[45] But these grand assertions were not based on experience or evidence as the IHDC made a point of asking for such and witnesses such as Mr Knyvett had to confess that 'I know of no case in which it has lead to temporary homicidal frenzy'.

---

[40] 'Report by Mr H. M. Lawrie CS Officiating Deputy Commissioner Bhandara, Central Provinces on the Consumption of Ganja among the Powars', ibid., iii. 240.
[41] 'Sind Memorandum', ibid., iii. 103.
[42] 'Bengal Memorandum', ibid., iii. 10–11.
[43] Ibid., i. 254.
[44] 'Evidence of Witnesses from North-Western Provinces and Oudh and Punjab', ibid., v. 109.
[45] 'Evidence of Bengal Witnesses', ibid., iv. 241.

The reason that the IHDC wanted evidence was that officers happily gave exciting conclusions that nevertheless, when challenged, went entirely without any supporting evidence. H. C. Williams, the magistrate of Darbhanga in Bengal, was called in front of the IHDC to flesh out his claim that cases of homicidal frenzy as a result of cannabis use were 'innumerable'. He was forced into a confession: 'my remark about cases of homicidal frenzy being innumerable is merely based on newspapers'.[46] Similarly, the Inspector-General of Police in the Central Provinces declared in his written statement that 'running "amok" is, I should say, always the result of excessive indulgence'. However, when hauled in front of the Commission and questioned on this declaration he had to concede that 'I have never had experience of such a case. I only state what I have heard.'[47] When one of his officers attempted to recall a case the result was hardly convincing.

The Balaghat case was about eighteen years ago. As far as I can remember, the criminal was a Banjara. He killed his own wife and two members of the tanda. It was not a case of jealousy; but I cannot say whether there was any cause of quarrel picked. I investigated the case as District Superintendent of Police. I remember ganja was alleged as the cause. My recollection is that he was convicted but I cannot be certain. It was above the Ghats. The man was probably also a liquor drinker for most Banjaras drink. He ran 'amok' with an axe. He had not, I think, been in that state before. He was placed under observation and my recollection is that he was held responsible for his act. But the people of the tanda alleged use of ganja as the cause of the outbreak. Many Banjaras (especially of the higher castes that do not drink) take ganja. I cannot say whether there had been any admixture in the ganja. Banjaras are a people rather given to violence.[48]

Indeed, so unconvinced by such bold assertions and such faltering evidence was the Commission that they chose to review all cases that their witnesses from across India cited as support for the argument that there was a connection between crime and the taking of cannabis preparations. It found that across India, of all of the rumours and half-remembered tales that were recounted, only 23 could be accurately located in the records. Having looked through the judicial papers on these cases, the Commission discovered that in only four cases could hemp substances safely be said to have caused the crime. The IHDC was staggered by its own finding and concluded that 'it is astonishing to find how defective and misleading are the recollections which many witnesses retain even of cases with which they

---

[46] 'Evidence of Bengal Witnesses', ibid., iv. 36.
[47] 'Evidence of Witnesses from Central Provinces and Madras', ibid., vi. 58–9.
[48] Ibid. 59.

have had special opportunities of being well acquainted. It is instructive to see how pre-conceived notions based on rumour and tradition tend to preserve the impression of certain particulars while the impressions of far more important features of the case are completely forgotten.' The IHDC was adamant in its conclusion, 'there is little or no connection between the use of hemp drugs and crime'.[49]

Given this problem of interpreting such a wealth of anecdotes, which were often unfounded and contradictory, the IHDC initiated a number of investigations of a scientific nature into cannabis. Bizarrely echoing the folk assumption mentioned above that cannabis had the effect of making the user look like a monkey, the IHDC directed Brigade-Surgeon Lieutenant Colonel Cunningham to begin work on a collection of the poor animals. The first chosen was a male *maccacus rhesus* that was subjected to the systematic inhalation of the smoke of ganja over eight months. In that time the monkey smoked ganja on 181 occasions, on an almost daily basis, explained the Brigade-Surgeon, except on Sundays and when the monkey had dysentery. The method of administering the smoke was to lock the animal inside a chamber that Cunningham very proudly detailed, as it was apparently one of his own devising. A chamber made of wooden walls coated in zinc, it had two plate glass windows for observation and tubes entering in the bottom of one side and the top of the other. The lower tube carried smoke from a chillum that was lit inside a glass bottle into the chamber and the higher tube was connected to a water-pump that drew the smoke through the box. Cunningham covered the joints in clay to ensure that there were not leaks and fretted only about residue gathering about the entrance of the in-tube.

The monkey, perhaps understandably, was at first reluctant to enter the Brigade-Surgeon's rather bizarre pride-and-joy and it seemed disturbed by the arrival of the smoke. Cunningham noted that 'the animal apparently disliked the treatment as he violently resisted introduction into the inhalation-chamber, was restless when the smoke began to enter it, and not unfrequently attempted to prevent its entrance by plugging the orifice of the tube'. A few days in with the fumes however seemed to have a remarkable effect on the subject of the experiment.

As time went on however and the experience lost its strangeness, his objections gradually diminished and were ultimately replaced by a positive desire for the treatment. He then readily entered the chamber, resisted any attempts to remove him from it before he had had a full dose, was restless and uneasy on days on

[49] Ibid., i. 263–4.

which the treatment was omitted, and on two occasions on which he managed to make his escape from his cage, showed an evident desire to enter the chamber on his own account.

Cunningham observed that the impact of the drug on the animal was to make him drowsy, unsteady on his legs, and eventually to put him to sleep. Upon waking, the animal seemed to have trouble focusing and the medical man suspected that he had some sorts of 'optical delusions' as he seemed to stare in directions where there was little to interest him. On a few occasions the monkey failed to go drowsy for a while and then suddenly was seized by convulsions upon which he fell profoundly unconscious. Cunningham could not make up his mind whether this was linked to variations in the quality of the drug or to peculiarities in the animal.

'In what but death, ends its sad tale?' went the Sindhi rhyme about cannabis use and this was all too true in this instance, although not for the reasons imagined by the poem's authors. Cunningham decided after eight months of getting the monkey stoned that he wanted to have a look at the physical impact of the drug on the animal's body, so he killed it and put it on the post-mortem slab. His main observation was there were large collections of fat on the omentum, the mesentery, and in the visceral and parietal pericardium. As the monkey had been given to eating less while caged, Cunningham reached the conclusion that smoking ganja may slow the processes of tissue waste in the body. As such, he made the point that in humans this would mean that those on poor diets undertaking hard work would benefit from smoking the drugs as it would slow the rate at which their bodies wore out. His experiments seemed to have identified a very important and beneficial effect of regular cannabis use.

It was a strange time to be an animal in Calcutta, as while Brigade-Surgeon Cunningham was entertaining his monkey to a smoke at the Zoological Garden, Surgeon-Captain J. F. Evans was feeding cannabis preparations to cats at his laboratories, provided that they were well behaved, that is 'fairly tame and docile, well nourished, and if females, not pregnant'. The 'tortoise-shell female cat' that was fed charas from Delhi was made of sterner stuff than the 'grey and white female cat' as the latter rocked and swayed while under the influence while the former was pencilled down as an 'effect nil'. The Nepal charas seemed not to be a feline favourite as it consistently scored an 'effect nil' but it appears that the Gurhwal charas was better as one cat became 'very much affected, is very unwilling to walk, and on being induced to move after a few steps falls over on its side'. On the whole, however, cats prefer bhang as the animal that was observed 'asleep with its nose on the ground' after almost five grains of the substance from Assam was by no means untypical. Ganja also had some impact on the subjects but it had the power to disturb the animals, as one cat was observed to be 'in distress and discomfort, pupils slightly dilated and the cat's appearance wild and suspicious; on being let loose the cat tries to hide itself', while another 'while apparently asleep with its eyes closed occasionally emitted a peculiar and unpleasant cry'.[50]

While the members of the IHDC initiated these experiments they also organized a review of that other set of 'scientific' data which had featured so prominently in debates about cannabis, the lunatic asylum statistics. They explicitly acknowledged the importance of these statistics in stirring up the whole debate about cannabis in the empire.

There has been undoubtedly a popular impression that hemp drugs do cause insanity ... besides this popular impression there has been great prominence given to asylum statistics as affording some tangible ground for judging of the effects of hemp drugs. Over and over again the statistics of Indian asylums have been referred to in official documents or scientific treatises not only in this country but also in other countries where the use of drugs has demanded attention.[51]

Indeed the Commission reiterated its belief in the influence of the numbers generated by the asylums in going as far as to say that 'hitherto any opinion regarding the connection between hemp drugs and insanity which has professed to have any solid basis at all or to be more than a vague impression has been based on the figures contained in the annual Statement no. VII appended to the Asylum reports'.[52] As such a comprehensive review of asylum practice and asylum records across the whole country was decided upon and the members of the Commission set off on a mammoth tour of the psychiatric system of India.

Every asylum in British India was visited either by the Commission or by some members of the Commission and careful enquiries were conducted on the spot in every case of insanity attributed to the use of hemp drugs for a given period. The period selected was the calendar year 1892, the last for which statistics were available at the commencement of the Commission's labours.[53]

---

[50] 'Report by Surgeon-Captain J. F. Evans, Chemical Examiner to the Government of Bengal, Regarding Physiological Investigations Concerning Hemp Drugs', ibid., iii. 206–27.
[51] 'Effects-Mental', ibid., i. 225.
[52] Ibid. 227.
[53] Ibid. 7.

The report identified the source of the information about the cause of the state of mind of the new admission supplied to the medical officers at the asylums.

The inquiry into the history of the case is not an inquiry conducted by a professional man from the persons likely to know most about the lunatic. The information consists often merely of the guesses of police officers as to the history and the habits of a friendless and homeless wanderer; and in other cases, where a local inquiry is possible, it is generally made by a subordinate police officer... It would be absurd to accept without great distrust the statements, especially as to the cause of insanity, compiled by such an agency as has been described.[54]

Those on the Commission also identified the forces acting on the police officers to make sure that the forms were correctly completed. They cited the example provided by a Commissioner of Excise in Assam[55] who recounted stories of instructions being issued to impose fines on subordinate police officers for failing to supply the necessary information. He also pointed to the action taken by Indian officials at the asylums who felt compelled to provide information where none was forthcoming: 'a striking illustration of the effect of this pressure is found in the Dullunda Asylum returns for the following year (1863) in which the cause in several cases dating from the year 1857 and onwards was later changed from "unknown" to "ganja-smoking" '.[56]

If the Commission discovered that the information being supplied to medical officers was coming from non-medical officers they also discovered that these medical officers were happy to believe this information. Surgeon-Major Willcocks at Agra provided the following testimony.

Ordinarily it has been the practice to enter hemp drugs as the cause of insanity where it has been shown that the patient used these drugs. I cannot say precisely why this is the practice. It has come down as the traditional practice. As a matter of fact until recently I looked upon these drugs as very poisonous. As I have already said, my ordinary medical practice did not bring me into contact with them at all. I only came into contact with them in the asylum. I had no idea that they were used as extensively as I find on enquiry to be the case.[57]

Dr Crombie of the Dacca asylum had published an article in the *Indian Medical Gazette* in 1892 that explained the statistical evidence of the asylums

---

[54] *Report of the IHDC*, iii. 231.
[55] Ibid. 232.
[56] Ibid.
[57] Ibid. 236.

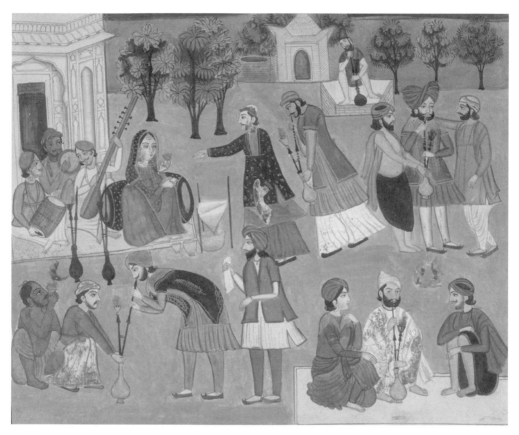

1. Gouache by Amritsar artist *c*.1870 depicting the smoking of Charras, a type of Indian hemp imported into northern India from Eastern Turkestan. The scene is a *Sakikhanâh* or charras shop. The woman on the left surrounded by minstrels is the seller or *Sâkan*. In other parts of the grounds of the *Sakikhanâh* different groups of smokers are represented. In the background a religious devotee is lazily imbibing the fumes of the drug. Just below to the right a native gentleman smokes while his servant holds the *hukkah* or smoking apparatus. The figure in the bottom right-hand corner is represented as coughing from the effects of the smoke. To his left the figure in the light-coloured turban is a seller (*saki*) who gives a few puffs of the drug for an *anna* or two. In the bottom left-hand corner a hindustani coolie or low-caste man is imbibing the fumes through his hands which he folds so as to act as a pipe to the earthen bowl in which Charras is burning. Archaeological Survey of India Collections: India Office Series (Volume 49). The painting accompanied samples of the narcotics illustrated, and was made for display at an unidentified exhibition.

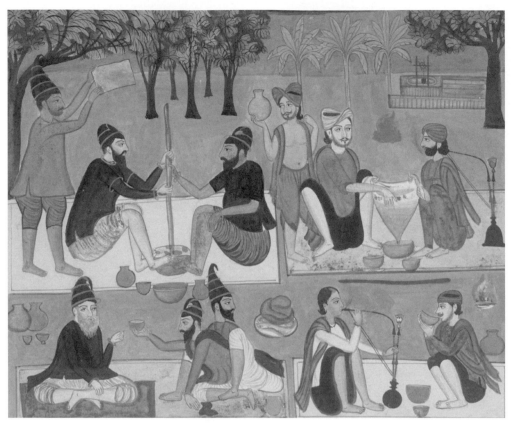

2. Gouache by Amritsar artist *c.*1870 depicting the preparation and consumption of Indian hemp (bhang). The men in black coats with circles of steel round their turbans are *akalis* or *nihangs*, a sect of Sikhs. The upper left-hand group represents the pounding of the leaves by *Sukhei*. To the right the preparation is being strained through cloth. Below two groups are represented as drinking the preparation. Archaeological Survey of India Collections: India Office Series (Volume 49). The painting accompanied samples of the narcotics illustrated, and was made for display at an unidentified exhibition.

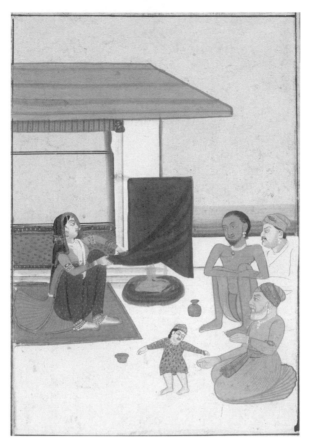

3. A woman straining bhang, a Faikier, a Borah, and a Hindu waiting to drink it. The picture depicts the idea that cannabis consumption transcended social distinctions in India. Anonymous, opaque watercolour *c*.1850, Rajasthan/Jaipur style.

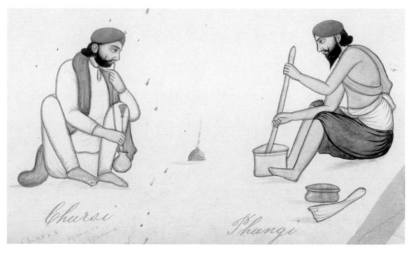

4. Men preparing and smoking Indian hemp. Anonymous watercolour, *c*.1860, Punjab style. The different artistic styles on this page reflect the fact that cannabis drugs were used across different regions and cultures in India.

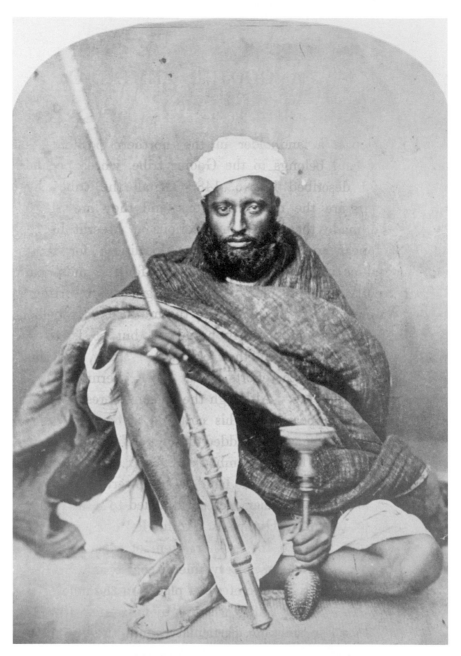

5. A zemindar. Goojur landholder, northern Saharunpoor district *c*.1860s. In his left hand is a hooka, the bottom of which is a coconut; into this a short stem of turned wood is inserted and the upper portion of chilum is made of pottery. The instrument is used either by a reed or tube of wood being placed into a hole in the coconut, or by applying the mouth to the orifice, which was by far the most usual method. J. Forbes Watson and John William Kaye, *The People of India. A Series of Photographic Illustrations with Descriptive Letterpress, of the Races and Tribes of Hindustan*, Volume III (India Museum, London, 1868).

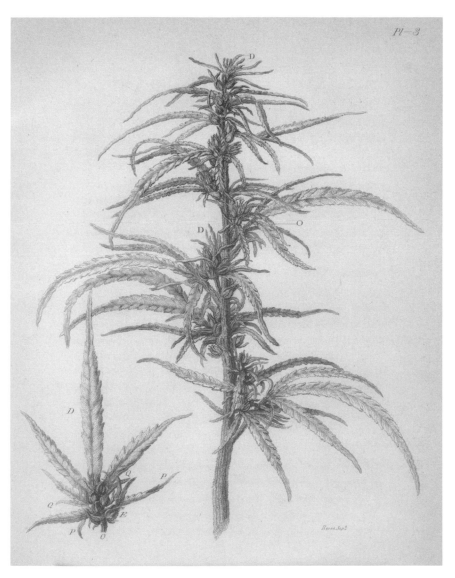

Pl - 3

6. A nineteenth-century sketch of the female cannabis plant in India. R. Wissett, *A Treatise on Hemp* (London, 1808). This book was typical of British interest in *cannabis sativa* in India in this period as it was preoccupied with schemes for cultivating the plant to be a source of fibres for naval rigging.

7. Portrait of the Reverend Thomas Evans. Evans was William Caine's companion on the latter's tour of India in 1889. He was also a committed temperance campaigner and a harsh critic of cannabis intoxicants in India. D. Hooper (ed.), *A Welshman in India: A Record of the Life of Thomas Evans, Missionary* (London, 1908).

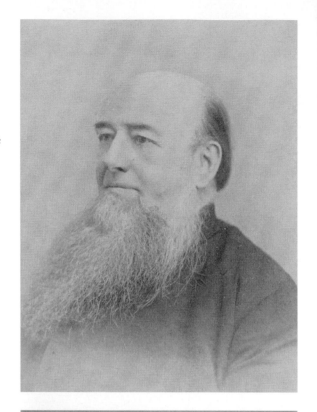

8. Portrait of William Sproston Caine MP. Caine mounted a one-man campaign against the Government of India on the issue of cannabis substances and secured the Indian Hemp Drugs Commission of 1893/4. J. Newton, *W. S. Caine, M.P.: A Biography* (London, 1907).

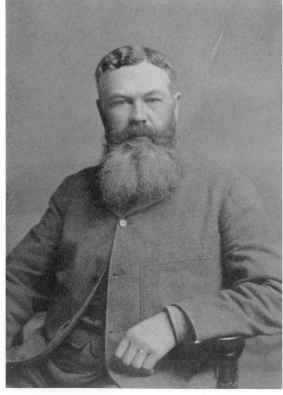

REPORT

OF THE

INDIAN HEMP DRUGS COMMISSION,

1893-94.

President :

The Hon'ble W. MACKWORTH YOUNG, M.A., C.S.I., First Financial Commissioner, Punjab.

Members :

1. Mr. H. T. OMMANNEY, Collector, Panch Mahals, Bombay.
2. Mr. A. H. L. FRASER, M.A., Commissioner, Chhattisgarh Division, Central Provinces.
3. Surgeon-Major C. J. H. WARDEN, Professor of Chemistry, Medical College, and Chemical Examiner to Government, Calcutta ; Officiating Medical Storekeeper to Government, Calcutta.
4. Raja SOSHI SIKHARESWAR ROY, of Tahirpur, Bengal.
5. KANWAR HARNAM SINGH, Ahluwalia, C.I.E., Punjab.
6. LALA NIHAL CHAND, of Muzaffarnagar, North-Western Provinces.

Secretary :

Mr. H. J. McINTOSH, Under-Secretary to the Government of Bengal, Financial and Municipal Departments.

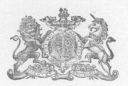

SIMLA|:
PRINTED AT THE GOVERNMENT CENTRAL PRINTING OFFICE.

1894.

9. Front page of the Report of the Indian Hemp Drugs Commission of 1894. This is the most extensive survey of a cannabis-using society by a Western government to date.

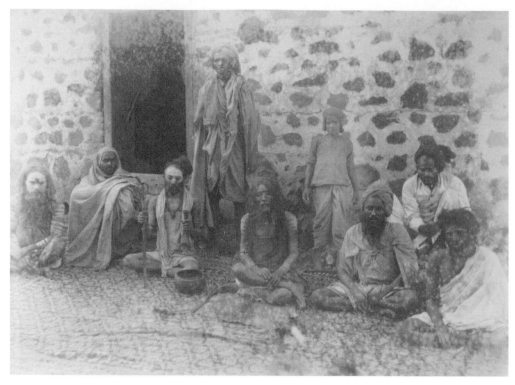

10. Group of Gossavis, habitual excessive ganja smokers, Khandesh. This photograph was taken for, and included in, the Report of the Indian Hemp Drugs Commission of 1894. It was one of a series depicting cannabis users who were grouped according to the frequency of use of the drug.

and showed how this proved that hemp drugs caused insanity. However he was forced by the Commission to agree that his conclusions were unreliable and admitted that his observations were almost entirely based on encounters in the asylum, 'in my practice outside of lunatic asylums my experience is confined to very few cases, only two or three in the whole course of my service, of ganja intoxication brought to hospital'.[58]

If the information coming in to the hospitals was difficult to believe then the statistics that were based on this information must also be questionable, decided the IHDC members. Indeed, they found that administrative interference or errors also tended to inflate the number of cannabis related cases. The report included an example to show where there were discrepancies between what was on the descriptive roll that accompanied the admission from the police or the magistrate and what was included on the asylum register: 'Dr Macnamara, Superintendent of the Tezpur Asylum says: "the cause is entered in the general register from the police statement i.e. from the descriptive roll. We have nothing whatever to do with it. It is entered by the Overseer in charge of the Asylum, and ought to correspond with the entry of the descriptive roll". As a matter of fact, eleven of the thirteen cases for 1892 showed entries regarding cause which did not correspond with the descriptive rolls; and of these 11, no less than 10 were made, not by the Overseer but by his subordinate, the jemedar'.[59] Similarly they reproduced an instance of apparent carelessness:

Moung Min Thay was admitted on 25th June 1871. There has been no improvement in his mental state. There are no papers in his case except an order from the Magistrate to receive the man 'supposed to be insane'. The original entry in the case book shows cause as 'predisposing disease of the brain, exciting drinks, and smokes opium', and it shows the duration as 'probably from birth'. It also shows that the man was epileptic. There is no mention of ganja. The register for 1885 (the first to show causation) shows 'alleged duration' as 'congenital' and 'alleged cause' as 'drink and opium smoking'. The entry 'congenital' is continued until 1892 when it is replaced by a 'Do' under the 'Not Given' of a previous case. In 1886 the 'cause' similarly undergoes undesigned alteration. The word 'drink' is replaced by 'ganja' and in 1888 the reference to 'opium' is finally dropped. The case thus became a ganja case, and has been shown as such ever since. These all may be instances of exceptional carelessness but as a general rule it cannot be said that these entries have been made with care. Superintendents have not attached much importance to them. It has been left to subordinates to do this work; and that work as a rule has not been carefully supervised.[60]

[58] Ibid. 234.   [59] Ibid.   [60] Ibid.

Indeed when the Commission went back through the records of those in the asylums who were admitted in 1892 they found that of the 222 cases across India attributed to use of cannabis only 98 could be regarded as in any way reliable. The Commission had acknowledged that the asylum statistics were an important factor in establishing a connection between hemp users, violence, and madness. However they were far from convinced that these statistics could be relied upon. In other words the final report of the IHDC concerned itself with exposing the process of categorization and enumeration which had lead to the establishment of the IHDC. It concluded that 'there was no trustworthy basis for a satisfactory and reasonably accurate opinion on the connection between hemp drugs and insanity in the asylum statistics appended to the annual reports'.[61]

THE CONCLUSIONS OF THE INDIAN HEMP DRUGS COMMISSION

After all of this work and all of this analysis the IHDC sat down to write the report. Once available, it had a number of important conclusions. It estimated that in Bengal about 1 in 200 consumed cannabis preparations and that of these users only about 5 per cent might be considered to be 'excessive' users. The annual consumption of a moderate user was established as 35 tolas (0.9 lb). The Central Provinces however were reckoned to be the region where cannabis users were most numerous but even there they only made up about 1 in 160 of the population. There appeared to be little evidence that use of the drugs was on the increase, although in areas where alcohol taxes had been increased, consumption of spirits had decreased while use of cannabis preparations had increased.

The IHDC stipulated that bhang was a harmless drink and that the government need have no worries about its use. It understood bhang to be a preparation of the leaves of the wild or cultivated plant that sometimes contained female flowering heads. It pointed out that there was often some confusion caused by the fact that bhang was also the name for fluid recipes of the drug. The majority of the IHDC reckoned that ganja was harmless if taken in moderation and they explained that ganja was made from the flowering tops of the female plants. Charas, however, was deemed to be more potent altogether as it was made from the resin exuded by the culti-

[61] '*Report of the IHDC*, iii. 237.

vated plants. It made the conclusion that as it was more powerful, charas must be more injurious to regular users.

Overall however the moderate use of the drugs was not felt to cause physical harm—'there is no evidence of any brain lesions being directly caused by hemp drugs as they have been found to be caused by alcohol and dhatura'[62]—and on the question of addiction the IHDC declared that 'the habit of using hemp drugs is easier to break off than the habit of using alcohol or opium'.[63] Indeed, they even offered the observation that 'it has been clearly established that the occasional use of hemp in moderate doses may be beneficial',[64] especially for those living in malarious regions and for those whose lives involved hard work or constant exposure. Excess, however, would lead to physical damage but they were keen to emphasize that this was the case with all intoxicants rather than just with hemp. Bronchitis and dysentery were the fate of those who indulged rather too freely.

The conclusions on the mental consequences of using hemp drugs were similarly attached to stipulations about moderate and excessive use. The IHDC declared that 'in respect to the alleged mental effects of the drugs, the Commission have come to the conclusion that the moderate use of hemp drugs produces no injurious effects on the mind'.[65] However, the IHDC also concluded that 'it appears that the excessive use of hemp drugs may, especially in cases where there is any weakness or hereditary predisposition, induce insanity'. Indeed, the desire to overindulge in these intoxicants was thought to be an indication of mental instability in the first place. The IHDC felt that it was important however to point to the conclusion of its extensive research into the nature of asylum statistics and popular impressions of the drug as it ended on the observation that 'it has been shown that the effect of hemp drugs in this respect has hitherto been greatly exaggerated'.[66]

As already stated, the IHDC felt that there were few social consequences of a population indulging in moderate doses of the drug. 'As a rule these drugs do not tend to crime and violence'[67] and even the excessive user was hardly likely to threaten public order except in the rarest of circumstances. Indeed, the report ended its round-up of the effects of the use of the drug with the following summary.

The large numbers of witnesses of all classes who professed never to have seen these effects, the vague statements made by many who professed to have observed them, the very few witnesses who could recall a case as to give any account of it, and the

[62] Ibid. 251.   [63] Ibid. 8.   [64] Ibid. 263.   [65] Ibid. 264.
[66] Ibid.   [67] Ibid. 258.

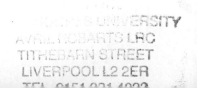

manner in which a large proportion of these cases broke down on the first attempt to examine them, are facts which combine to show most clearly how little injury society has hitherto sustained from hemp drugs.[68]

As this was the case, the IHDC approached the question of prohibiting the use of the drugs very cautiously. Quoting precedents from 1798, 1872, and 1892, it pointed out that prohibition had been considered at various times over the last century of British rule in India and that it had always been rejected. The grounds for this rejection was that the plant grew wild and that therefore it would be difficult to stop preparation of drugs from these natural sources and that any attempt to stop such a common habit threatened both to provoke the local population and to force them into using more damaging intoxicants.

To these grounds the IHDC added others. First of all, it asserted that as bhang, ganja, and charas were relatively harmless to moderate consumers and as it had established that there were no social problems attendant on its use there was no case for prohibition. Secondly, it produced a philosophical defence of its decision to reject prohibition as it extensively quoted J. S. Mill's theories of political economy:

To be prevented from what one is inclined to, or from acting contrary to one's own judgement of what is desirable, is not only always irksome, but always tends pro tanto to starve the development of some portion of the bodily or mental faculties, either sensitive or active; and unless the conscience of the individual goes freely with the legal restraint, it partakes either in a great or in a small degree of the degradation of slavery. Scarcely any degree of utility short of absolute necessity will justify a prohibitory regulation, unless it can be made to recommend itself to the general conscience.[69]

Rather than prohibit, the IHDC decided that the government ought to do nothing to promote moderate use and ought to positively discourage excessive use, while at the same time refraining from any measure that might encourage smuggling or force consumers to turn to other, more dangerous substances. The IHDC's recommendations were therefore aimed at standardization of hemp taxation policy in India rather than at a radical overhaul that would have come with a demand for prohibition. 'The policy advocated is one of control and restriction' argued the IHDC and it decided that four main planks of policy needed to be adopted—'adequate taxation', 'prohibiting cultivation except under licence', 'limiting the

[68] *Report of the IHDC*, iii. 264.
[69] Ibid. 266.

number of shops', and 'limiting the extent of legal possession'. Most important of all 'the method adopted should be systematic and as far as possible uniform for the whole of British India and . . . certain of the Native States'.[70] Bengal was to be the model, and the IHDC was in favour of limits on the amount that any individual could possess.

POLITICAL AGENDAS AND INDIAN DISSENTERS

If this chapter argued earlier that the origins of the orders to establish the IHDC were mired in the politics of Britain's drug trade in Asia and of its colonial rule in India then it also suggests that it is difficult to avoid the suspicion that the conclusions of its report had their roots in specific interests within the empire. This becomes apparent when the reactions to the dissenters from within the members of the IHDC itself are considered. The dissenters from the conclusions of the IHDC were Indian, Raja Soshi Sikareshwar Ray and Lala Nihal Chand both entering lengthy notes into the report that stated that they were far from in agreement with various of the conclusions. Ray made it clear that 'I believe that the injurious effects of the hemp drugs are greater and their use more harmful than one would naturally suppose to be the case after reading the concluding portion of Chapter XIII of our Report, although I think I should say that the facts elicited by our inquiry do not go to support the extreme opinion held by some well-intentioned people that these drugs in all their forms and in every case are highly pernicious in their effects.'[71] He went on to explain that he felt that the drugs had physically debilitating effects on the poorly nourished in a very short time and even in cases of relatively moderate usage. It was just this issue that the results of Brigade-Surgeon Cunningham's experiments with the monkeys had dealt with as he had concluded that certain preparations were actually physically beneficial to the poorly fed and hard working. It is important to bear in mind, however, that Cunningham's experiments were conducted as an employee of the government zoo in Calcutta, the capital of Bengal, the Presidency that profited most from cannabis use in Indian society.

Lala Nihal Chand's objection to the IHDC's report was that there was plenty of evidence in the witness statements that profoundly contradicted the conclusions settled upon by the Commission. He went through the witness

70 Ibid. 359.
71 'Resolution of Finance and Commerce Department', ibid. 12.

statements and listed at length those that disagreed with the IHDC's broad conclusions. He then disputed the IHDC's hatchet job on the lunatic asylum statistics, complaining that 'as will be seen from paragraph 521 of the Report, out of 222 ganja cases 124 have been rejected. In my opinion many of them have been rejected on insufficient grounds.'[72] He was in favour of prohibiting charas and ganja consumption in the long term, and as an immediate measure he wanted a register of users of hemp drugs to be drawn up as the beginnings of a surveillance system designed to keep tabs on this group of 'bad characters, low class people, and beggars'.[73]

These objections were swept aside by the Governor-General's Resolution on the Commission. Raja Soshi Sikareshwar Ray was rather patronizingly chided with the laissez-faire logic that 'there are many matters in which adults must be allowed to judge for themselves'.[74] Lala Nihal Chand had been absent for much of the second tour of the Commission and this was used to discredit his objections. The Finance and Commerce Department was also careful to dispute his arguments and produced a whole set of witness statements from the IHDC to refute each of his points which it appended to the Resolution.[75] The Department, whose Excise section managed the hefty annual income from the taxation of cannabis drugs in India, went to some effort in order to defend the sympathetic conclusions of the IHDC.

The Governor-General also wrote enthusiastically in support of the IHDC's recommendations:

The Governor General in Council must observe that even accepting to the full the Raja's estimate of the evidence as to the injurious nature of ganja and its possible confirmation by future enquiries, he cannot consider that prohibition would become the duty of Government or would even be justifiable. There are many matters in which adults must be allowed to judge for themselves and to use their own discretion and the mere fact that some of them would be benefited, morally or physically, by abstention from any particular indulgence does not warrant the Government in making that indulgence penal. For it is beyond a doubt that it is only by attaching to the cultivation, or sale of hemp drugs, the penalties of the criminal law, that prohibition could be made effective.[76]

---

[72] 'Note of Dissent by Lala Nihal Chand', ibid. 417.

[73] Ibid. 436.

[74] 'Resolution of Finance and Commerce Department', ibid 13.

[75] Appendix to the 'Resolution of Finance and Commerce Department: Examination of the Evidence Quoted in Lala Nihal Chand's Minute of Dissent', ibid.

[76] 'Resolution of Finance and Commerce Department', ibid. 13.

absurdities of the most grotesque kind, leaping, beating time to nothing, moving their arms as if receiving electrical shocks, writing ridiculous words and feeling as if they were independent of the acts.

The article left little doubt that 'the peculiar intoxication induced by the narcotic is certainly destructive to sound mental life'.[5] If this were not shocking enough for the reader of *Abkari* a couple of pages later he or she would have discovered, thanks to the Reverend Thomas Evans, that his or her fellow countrymen in government in India were in fact the overlords of 'the State traffic in the noxious ganja poison'.[6] This was followed in the October issue by a reprint of an article from the *Times of India* which referred to Sir William Hunter's warning to anti-opiumists that restrictions on the use of that drug would drive people to 'one much more pernicious', that is the dreaded ganja. The campaign on cannabis in the *Abkari* really got going, however, to correspond with William Caine's agitations in Parliament. The April 1893 issue devoted three articles to hemp drugs—a 'Notes on Ganja', a piece written by 'An ex-Commissioner of Bengal on Indian Hemp', and a list of 'Regulations affecting the Importation and Sale of Haschisch'. The latter was a list of countries where there were already regulations dealing with cannabis preparations which will be discussed separately in Chapter 7 as it was in fact a reprint of an India Office report. Brigade-Surgeon R. Pringle presented the 'Notes on Ganja' and conjured up images of the heathen guaranteed to shock his largely Christian audience: 'the terrible wrecks of humanity, seen in the cases of many devotees at the sacred shrines in Bengal, such as Juggernauth, Hurdwar etc... are fearful illustrations of the awful effects of the cultivation, production and the sale of a poisonous drug carried on under a special licence from the Government'.[7] The fact that the devotees that he described preferred lean bodies as a sign of their asceticism and consumed cannabis as part of their spiritual exercises seems not to have occurred to the Brigade-Surgeon.

[5] B. W. Richardson, 'Indian Hemp as an Intoxicant', ibid. 3 (1892), 9–10.
[6] T. Evans, 'The Cultivation of "Ganja" by the Indian Government', ibid. 3 (1892), 14–17. Evans was a Welsh Baptist missionary in India who had been in the country since 1855. He took to sending letters to the British newspapers and it was these that drew him to the attention of MPs in the House of Commons who shared his concern with the issues of temperance, the opium trade, and the government of India. William Caine contacted him in the summer of 1888 and invited Evans to accompany him on a tour of India, on which they spoke to almost a hundred temperance meetings in most of the key cities of British India. Evans believed that 'the indulgence in opium is bad enough, but not half as injurious as that of ganja' (*Report of the IHDC*, v. 304) and it therefore seems that he was chief among those responsible for sparking William Caine's interest in cannabis substances, and for convincing him of the case against them.
[7] 'Notes on Ganja', ibid. 13 (Apr. 1893), 58.

The article by J. Monro, formerly a Commissioner in Bengal and Chief Commissioner of Police in London, was similarly concerned to create anxieties about cannabis use in India. He produced statistics from the lunatic asylums of Bengal to make his case, the statistics that seem so problematic in light of the evidence in Chapters 4 and 5. He also declared that the government took revenue of almost £150,000 per annum from duties on the trade in cannabis, which rather took the sting out of Brigade-Surgeon Pringle's somewhat more audacious claim in the same issue that this sum was in fact 'nearly a quarter of a million sterling'.[8] Monro assured readers that 'unlike opium, which is a sedative, ganja is of a highly exciting nature; it stimulates the brain and renders its victims reckless, furious, mad'.[9]

The focus of *Abkari* on the cannabis issue continued during the operations of the IHDC and the 3,000 copies of each quarterly issue drew attention to the subject as it circulated around the 131 societies in Britain and India that had affiliated to the Anglo-Indian Temperance Associations by 1893.[10] It is difficult to tell exactly how many people came to see the issues of the magazine but beyond those who actually had the opportunity to thumb through a copy it seems that others became aware of its contents as they were reproduced elsewhere and for other audiences: 'it is largely quoted by the Indian press and the constant translation of its articles into the vernacular for gratuitous circulation by our branches are gratifying evidence of its value to our movement'.[11] Those that had contact with the reporting in one of its many forms would have been assured throughout 1893–4 that adding cannabis to the local liquor 'drives the British soldier mad, and leads him to commit suicide or as I know, the most carefully planned and cold-blooded murder',[12] that ganja smokers found that 'the mind gets full of horrible imaginations',[13] and that the drugs in general 'tend to insanity and homicidal mania'.[14]

However, the articles on hemp drugs dried up upon the release of the report of the IHDC. Nothing appeared in the October 1894 issue except the news that the *Times of India* claimed to have seen the report by 31 August 1894. The January 1895 edition was full of portraits of the good

    [8] 'Notes on Ganja', ibid. 13 (Apr. 1893), 58.
    [9] 'An ex-Commissioner of Bengal on Indian Hemp', ibid. 13 (Apr. 1893), 71.
    [10] 'Annual Report 1892–3', ibid. 14 (July 1893), 109.
    [11] Ibid.
    [12] 'Indian Hemp from a Public Health Point of View', ibid. 14 (1893), 120.
    [13] 'Hemp Drugs in Bengal', ibid. 16 (1894), 14.
    [14] 'Hemp Drugs', ibid. 18 (1894), 93.

and the great of the Anglo-Indian Temperance Association, the April issue stated only that William Caine had asked after the IHDC report in Parliament, and in October it was simply mentioned that he had received the report. Indeed, the only pages devoted to the issue of the IHDC report thereafter were a three-page bleat about government bias penned by Joshua Rowntree, who had similarly attacked the Opium Commission.[15] This was tucked away in William Caine's editorial section of the magazine titled 'Current Notes'. Rowntree complained about the influence of the Indian government over the IHDC before quibbling about the definition of 'moderate use' in the IHDC's conclusions. Typical of the piece is the important observation that at one point in the report it noted that excessive use was 'most exceptional' while later it was deemed to be only 'exceptional'. Indeed, Rowntree promised a further report on the IHDC in the next issue. This never materialized and in fact *Abkari* failed to devote a single article thereafter to the issue of hemp at any point before the death of Caine in 1903, despite having twelve pieces on the subject between 1892 and 1894. Caine himself never used the space available to him in the journal to renew the campaign against cannabis. The issue of hemp drugs was quickly forgotten by the temperance campaigners once the IHDC challenged their assumptions and assertions. *Abkari* and its members took comfort in turning their attention to the other perceived evils of the colonial government such as its dealings in alcohol in India.

GOVERNMENT AND THE INDIAN HEMP DRUGS COMMISSION REPORT

While the IHDC failed to excite much attention in British politics or in temperance or anti-opium circles it similarly failed to have a sudden and significant impact in India. Alongside its general observations that adequate taxation, prohibition of unlicensed cultivation, a limitation on the number of shops, and a restriction on personal possession were the fundamentals of hemp policy, the Commission made a number of more detailed recommendations.

That in Bengal Government warehouses for the storage of ganja should be constructed in Rajshahi.

---

[15] J. Rowntree, *The Opium Habit in the East: A Study of the Evidence Given to the Royal Commission on Opium 1893/4* (King, London, 1895).

That subject to this addition, the Bengal system of ganja administration should be generally followed in the Central Provinces, Madras, Bombay, Berar and possibly in Ajmere and Coorg.

That the limit of legal possession of the hemp drugs should be the same for the whole of British India viz Ganja and charas, or any preparation or admixture thereof, 5 tolas, bhang or any preparation or admixture thereof, one quarter of a ser. And that Native States should be invited to adopt this maximum.[16]

It seems, however, that measures designed to make local governments comply with the IHDC recommendations were in fact adopted in a reluctant manner. The states of Berar were specifically named in the above recommendations of the IHDC. These states were a cause for concern as they nestled between the Central Provinces and the Bombay Presidency and because they levied no direct customs on their hemp. Indeed as early as 1888 they had been identified as a problem and 'the Chief Commissioner [of the Central Provinces] authorized the Commissioner of Excise to consult the Commissioner of Berar with regard to the cultivation of ganja in that province and the possibility of checking its carriage across the Central Provinces border'.[17] Yet Berar was hardly energetic in carrying into effect the recommendations of the IHDC as it took the British Resident over three years to get around to putting legislation in place. In November 1897 he decided that he was 'pleased to issue the following orders to make better provision for the production, sale, possession and import of intoxicating drugs and for the collection of revenue therefrom in the Hyd. Assigned Districts'.[18] These orders empowered the Resident to make a number of decisions about the Indian hemp drugs trade. For instance, the Resident could now if he so decided

prohibit absolutely or except under and subject to conditions of a license granted by such officers as the Resident may from time to time appoint in his behalf, the cultivation of the hemp plant and the preparation or production of intoxicating drugs from the hemp plant so cultivated and place the cultivation of the hemp plant and the production or preparation and storage of such intoxicating drugs as aforesaid under such supervision as may be deemed necessary to secure payment of duty (if any) imposed under this Law.[19]

Indeed, the Berar Hemp Drugs Law also gave the Resident the power to control the transport of prepared drugs, the import of hemp drugs into his

---

[16] *Report of the Indian Hemp Drugs Commission 1893–4* (Simla, 1894), i. 360–1.

[17] 'Central Provinces Memorandum', ibid., iii. 72.

[18] Foreign Department, Berar Hemp Drugs Law 1897 and rules issued thereunder.

[19] Ibid.

region, and even to 'restrict and regulate' the amount of drugs that the locals could prepare from the wild hemp growing on the verges and in their paddocks. He was given the power to erect a system of government ware-houses for storing the prepared drugs and was enabled to levy duty on these products. Perhaps most importantly he was given powers over consumers as well as producers. Nobody was allowed to possess more than one seer of bhang or five tolas of ganja or charas unless they had a licence to do so. If someone was suspected of carrying more than this in their possession then they risked ruin and the wrath of the Customs officers: 'any Excise officer may stop and detain any person carrying any intoxicating drug liable to confiscation under this Law and may seize such drug together with any vessels, packages or coverings in which it is contained and any animals and conveyances used in carrying it and may also arrest the person in whose possession such drug is found'.[20] Indeed, the state gave itself the right not simply to harass people out on the highways but to violently intervene in the households and workplaces of the local communities.

Such officer may, after sunrise and before sunset (but always in the presence of an officer of police not below the rank of head Constable unless the Excise Officer is himself such an officer of police) enter into such a place and in case of resistance may break open any door and force and remove any other obstacle to such entry and may seize and carry away such article and may also arrest the occupier of the place with all other persons concerned in the keeping and concealing of such an article.

Although it took three years for the Berar government to get around to developing these regulations they were severe in contrast with what had gone on before. In previous regulations 'there [was] nothing laid down as to the amount of possession' and the only surveillance that was operated was of the retail vendors whose 'shops are occasionally inspected by officers'.[21]

Meanwhile in Bengal, which the IHDC had recommended as the model for the rest of India, there were considerable delays in erecting the public warehouses as advocated by the Commission and only slow im-provements in other aspects of the system. A report of 1904 compiled by G. Rainy, a British Magistrate on special duty, on the 'manufacture and smuggling of ganja' despaired that

From 1894 10 per cent of the fields were measured with ropes by the Assistant Supervisors but there was no check on their measurements.

---

[20] Ibid.   [21] 'Berar Memorandum' in *Report of the IHDC*, iii. 112–3.

In 1895 the Bengal Government resolved to erect public warehouses at Naugaon for the storage of the drug.

In 1896 the outturn was for the first time actually weighed in the chattars before storage.

In 1902–03 an improved scheme was introduced by which ten per cent of the fields were measured by the Assistant Supers with Gunter's chain and optical right angle and 20 percent of their work checked by the Sub Deputy Collector.

In 1904 for the first time the whole of the crop was stored in the public golas from the chattar.

Up till 1903 the cultivators were allowed the option of storing privately up to a certain date when part of the crop having been exported the remainder could be accommodated in the public golas. Even in the present year the gola accommodation is quite insufficient and it has only been possible to store the whole of the crop by taxing the storage accommodation to the utmost.[22]

In other words, in that province where the administration of hemp narcotics had traditionally been most efficient it had still taken almost ten years from the time of the IHDC for the government to erect enough warehouses to store the crop in order to ensure an accurate assessment of the amount of drugs that were about to enter the system. However the author of the report was still far from convinced that even these measures had managed to stamp out smuggling. He wished to expand the Ganja Supervisor's Office once again to include a new cadre of Deputy Inspectors to keep an eye on the Indian officers that were patrolling the hemp districts. However, in times of harvest he intended to have the entire policing system of Bengal involved with the business of ganja smuggling. He suggested first of all that 'the Railway authorities and the Railway Police may be fairly asked to cooperate with the Excise Department to prevent the smuggling of ganja by rail'. Then he suggested that 'the second thing is this, that all Excise Officers, Police officers, and chaukidars [village watchmen] in the districts of Bogra, Dinajpur and Rajshahi should be instructed to be on the alert during the manufacturing season and give the earliest possible information of any suspected smuggling'. However, the village watchmen were not simply to keep an eye out for smuggling in their district, they were to be employed in the processes of prevention.

The services of the chaukidars can also be utilised in another way, namely for the surveillance of convicted ganja smugglers. Every person previously convicted of

[22] G. Rainy, *Report on the Manufacture and Smuggling of Ganja* (Bengal Secretariat Press, Calcutta, 1904), 9.

ganja smuggling and resident in any village in the district of Bogra, Dinajpur or Rajshahi outside the ganja mahal should be kept under constant surveillance during the manufacturing season. The village chaukidar should be required to visit his house twice every night during February and March and if he is found absent the chaukidar should be required to report the fact at the thana as early as possible the next day. The thana officer should be instructed to report the fact direct to the SubDivisional Officer at Naugaon without delay. This will enable the Excise officers to follow in some degree the movements of convicted smugglers and to keep a watch for them.[23]

When Hem Chunder Kerr had reported on hemp drugs administration back in the 1870s the supervision of the drugs trade had been the business of a dozen or so Excise officers. Thirty years later it was envisaged that all of the police squads of eastern Bengal ought to be involved in systems of surveillance and detection.

Perhaps the most dilatory of the administrations in India regarding the recommendations of the IHDC was that of Bombay. It did not get round to limiting personal possession of ganja and bhang until 1913, almost twenty years after the establishment of the Commission. Indeed, these limits were finally imposed not because of any sense of sudden urgency about the issue of cannabis preparations but because of a determination to control the growing cocaine problem among the people of the city. Albert Niemann extracted the primary alkaloid from coca leaves in 1859 and named it cocaine. It was soon heralded as a wonder-drug and Freud, Thomas Edison, and Pope Leo XIII were among the enthusiasts for various preparations of cocaine, which, perhaps most famously, was the key ingredient in the original recipe for Coca-Cola.[24] Such was the popularity of the substance for a period that the British in India, never slow to try out new money-making ideas, actively encouraged Indian farmers to grow coca crops in parts of Assam and Madras. Indeed, it was reported that 'experiments in this direction were made with some success'.[25] However, by 1887 Freud had published 'Craving for and Fear of Cocaine' and stories of addiction to the drug and of mental health problems and even of deaths that were a result of its use became common. Throughout the first decades of the twentieth century legislation began to limit public access to the drug, so that in the USA the 1914 Harrison Act made cocaine substances

[23] Ibid. 30.

[24] See M. Gold, *Cocaine* (Plenum, London, 1993), 13–15.

[25] From GOI (Excise) to Government of Bombay (Revenue) 4 May 1911, in Bombay General File 1913/100.

available only on medical prescription and in 1916 the British government made possession of the drug illegal unless for medical purposes.[26]

Interestingly, the British in India seem to have been unusually concerned with the issue of cocaine as the first steps towards regulating its usage were made in Bombay in 1903, a date that preceded the earliest American regulation (in New York State) by three years. In Bombay it was stipulated that sale of the drug would be allowed only for medical purposes and that only those chemists and doctors with a licence to sell the drug would be legally entitled to do so. However, it seems that alongside this law there remained the right to possess up to one-tenth of a grain of cocaine whatever the status of the individual. This ensured enough of a loophole in the law for the entrepreneurial cocaine dealers of the city. Under these laws they could only be arrested for carrying or supplying the drug where it could be proved that what they carried or sold contained more than one-tenth of a grain.

Their key means of getting around the laws then was to supply cocaine in a form that made the substance difficult to isolate and measure in chemical analysis.

The cocaine hawkers of Bombay have now commenced to sell betel leaves on which has been smeared cocaine mixed with lime with the result that it will be impossible in most such cases to ascertain whether the amount of cocaine on the leaf is or is not in excess of one tenth of a grain.[27]

This had all come to light as the government had arrested one such hawker and sent him off to be prosecuted. The evidence of the Chemical Analyser was of course crucial as only he could determine whether the substance that the hawker was selling was in breach of the one-tenth of a grain regulation. He declared that 'I have the honour to state that the analysis of the smeared leaves showed the presence of 0.26 grains of an alkaloidal or quasi-alkaloidal substance which contained cocaine. The determination of the exact proportion of cocaine present in such a product is not a very satisfactory operation. I am not prepared to state definitely that the figure given represents the quantity of cocaine present.'[28] The accused was acquitted.

[26] Gold, *Cocaine*, 17; V. Berridge, 'War Conditions and Narcotics Control: The Passing of Defence of the Realm Act Regulation 40B', *Journal of Social Policy*, 7/3 (1978), 285–304.
[27] From General Department to Revenue Department 16 May 1913, in Bombay General File 1913/100.
[28] From Chemical Analyser to Assistant Collector of Excise Bombay 11 April 1913, ibid.

The hawker's approach was ingenious as the use of a betel leaf as a container for various sweetmeats and refreshers was an everyday practice and was as common in India then as it is today. As this was the case the vendor would have made himself inconspicuous in market-places by using such leaves alongside ones smeared with less narcotic mixtures and he would have been administering the drug in a way that would have been familiar to his customers. The government fretted that after the man's acquittal 'the decision is now widely known among the cocaine hawkers and the practice of smearing cocaine on betel leaves with the object of defeating a quantitative analysis is sure to spread'.[29]

The reason that cocaine could be possessed in even the small amount of one-tenth of a grain, and indeed the reason for the failure of the government in Bombay to impose restrictions on the amount of cannabis that an individual could carry, lay in the old customs laws of 1878. They needed to be overhauled in their entirety in order to facilitate proper limitations. These were finally revised in 1912 so the issue of the possession of drugs was raised in light of the urgency of combating the cocaine hawkers who had just found a way around prosecution. Possession of 'Coca leaves, alkaloids of coca, every other intoxicating drink or substance prepared from the coca plant (erythroxylum coca) and all drugs, synthetic or other, having a like physiological effects to that of cocaine' in any amount was prohibited for all except licensed medical practitioners. The reform of the customs laws also gave the government of Bombay the opportunity to bring its regulations on other intoxicants into line with the rest of India so that it imposed restrictions on liquor, toddy, and Indian hemp. Individuals were allowed to carry only 5 tolas of ganja, 3 tolas of charas, and 20 tolas of bhang at any one time.[30]

The striking feature of the reports of this period after the IHDC, and indeed of British rule in India as a whole, is that whatever the deliberations of the Government of India and the interest in the subject of the House of Commons and no matter how much policy was devised and implemented Indians continued to produce and to consume cannabis products in sizeable quantities. The producers of the Ganja Mahal, one of the oldest regions of hemp production in India that was detailed by Hem Chunder Kerr as early as the 1870s, seemed to continue making their fortunes from the trade in hemp drugs. G. Rainy observed in 1903, almost ten years after the report of the IHDC, that the cultivators in the region were 'without doubt the richest and most prosperous body of peasantry in Bengal and

[29] From General Department to Revenue Department 16 May 1913, ibid.
[30] Revenue Department Order 6706E 21 July 1913, ibid.

their wealth and prosperity is the direct gift of Government, which has made them its partners in an enormously valuable monopoly'. In order to back up this rather grand claim he provided a couple of anecdotal instances to prove what he said.

When the Excise Commissioner visited Naugaon in 1903 a proposal was on foot to export a large quantity of ganja to Madras where the supply was short. The proposal came to nothing but when it was entertained it was found that it would be necessary to raise Rs 60000 at short notice to finance the export. One of the cultivators Jarif Mandal was summoned to Naugaon and asked whether the money could be raised. His answer was that although he had not the money himself he was prepared to get it from his mother and produce it the same day. This man is probably the richest of all the cultivators but not by a very great deal; there are others that are not much his inferiors. The ganja cultivators contributed amongst them Rs 5000 for the creation of the Higher English School at Naugaon. If a road or a bridge is wanted, instead of waiting for the tardy action of a District Board or committing themselves to the tender mercies of the PWD the cultivators raise a subscription among themselves and the road or bridge is constructed.[31]

Indeed, the British magistrate and the cannabis cultivators seemed to have had a very cosy view of one another and a very amicable relationship as Rainy went on to eulogize: 'They are singularly peaceable and law abiding and they are remarkably wealthy and prosperous. The impression they created on my mind was a most favourable one. I found them uniformly pleasant to deal with, frank without bumptiousness and courteous without servility.'

It was certainly the case that while the producers were prospering, the government, for all of the bluster in the IHDC about using taxation to control consumption, was happily sharing in the money to be made from cannabis use. The 'Memorandum on Excise Administration in India so far as it is concerned with Hemp Drugs' tracked the revenue raised from cannabis preparations from 1900 onwards. In that year it was discovered that the British in India raised taxes worth 5,564,000 rupees on the cannabis drugs trade across their territories in South Asia. Of this 2,790,000 was raised in Bengal alone where revenue from hemp drugs levies made up a startling one-fifth of the total excise income for the year. In that region 3.2 seers of cannabis preparations were consumed per thousand people every year (a seer weighed the equivalent of about 2 imperial pounds).[32] Five

---

[31] Rainy, *Report on Ganja*, 23.
[32] Memorandum on Excise Administration in India so far as it is concerned with Hemp Drugs (Simla Government Printing Office, 1901), 21–2.

years later the figures showed that there had actually been an increase in these figures. The British now took Rs 7,786,000 in revenue from the trade. In Bengal consumption was now almost 4 seers per thousand of the population.[33] The next report that is available is for the year 1921, and this shows that in the space of two decades little had changed. In Bengal revenue from hemp drugs still accounted for about a fifth of the total excise receipts but in Bihar and Orissa, a new state that had been hived off from the old Bengal Presidency in 1911, it amounted to over a quarter of the revenue. In the new capital city, Delhi, the tax on hemp narcotics made up a third of all excise income. Consumption in Bengal and in Bihar and Orissa had dropped from almost 4 seers per thousand of the population in 1905 to about 2.5 seers per head of the population. Across the country however, total revenue now amounted to Rs 18,347,000.[34]

Use of hemp drugs in the immediate aftermath of the IHDC seems therefore to have shown no signs of abating and in a number of the provinces for which there is evidence consumption seems to have actually been on the increase. In Assam for example, there was an 88 per cent increase in consumption of cannabis preparations between 1901 and 1911 and this was far in excess of any increase in population. The government at first blamed the labouring population in the region that was not indigenous but went there to work on the plantations; 'good times and higher wages on the tea gardens are doubtless also responsible for a portion of the increase'.[35] But it was pointed out that while consumption had gone up by such a percentage the increase in the immigrant labouring population had only gone up by 34 per cent so it was unlikely that the coolies could alone account for the massive rise. The report of the Committee appointed to inquire into aspects of opium and ganja consumption in 1913 in Assam found that all manner of groups had taken to ganja smoking. The local cultivators, the boatmen, and the river-borne traders took to the habit and the report pointed out that 'the excuse given by them is that the drug assists them to bear fatigue and exposure'. The lower castes such as the Nadials, Charals, and Hiras similarly claimed such reasons for using the drug and the Committee discovered that consumption 'has also been very marked amongst the higher castes, who take it purely as a luxury'. Indeed, it

[33] Memorandum on Excise Administration in India so far as it is concerned with Hemp Drugs (Simla Government Printing Office, 1906), 24.

[34] Memorandum on Excise Administration in India so far as it is concerned with Hemp Drugs (Simla Government Printing Office, 1922), 18–19.

[35] 'The Report of the Committee Appointed to Enquire into Certain Aspects of Opium and Ganja Consumption', *Assam Gazette*, 10 Dec. 1918, 1586.

appears that ganja smoking could also now be found in the religious activities of the regions whereas previously it had been opium that played a role in *Namgaos* religious services and such festivals as those connected with a marriage. The report observed the 'influence of the numbers of up-country or Bengali sanyasis who pass through the district on the way to Kamakhya. One of these gentry in particular appears to have established a regular cult of ganja smokers in the neighbourhood of Nalbari.'[36]

The reason for the number of new consumers and for the spread of consumption through all parts of society in Assam lay in the relative expense of opium compared to ganja and in the growing awareness of the health problems associated with use of preparations of the poppy. 'Opium consumption is going down in my mauza because knowing the evil effects of opium people are taking to ganja', observed one officer. All manner of solutions were suggested to tackle this growing drug consumption in the region. As usual an increase in duty was suggested as a means of discouraging consumption by making the product more expensive for the consumer, especially as the report found that the price of hemp preparations had not increased in Assam since the 1890s whereas there had been a steady rise in the cost of living in general. It was suggested that the maximum that any one individual could own be reduced to 5 tolas, which points to the fact that almost twenty years after the IHDC Assam had failed to implement its recommendations on possession. Interestingly, there seems to be no awareness of the IHDC anywhere in the report while there is at least a passing reference to the Opium Commission.[37] Another suggestion that the Assam Committee came up with was that the age at which consumers could take to ganja was to be raised to 20 from the current age of 10 in order to attempt to discourage new customers for the drug.

It was feared, however, that any state imposed restrictions were unlikely to have much effect while there was a demand for the drug as wild hemp grew so freely on the fertile soils of Assam. The Committee heard witnesses who were certain that 'wild ganja is smoked more than excise ganja in my village as well as in other villages. All castes of Hindus, including Kalitas, Brahmins and others smoke wild ganja. There is hardly any villager who does not smoke wild bhang in my village.' Others noted a relationship between the excise and wild products, and one local testified that 'if they cannot get excise ganja some smoke wild bhang. I have smoked wild

[36] 'The Report of the Committee Appointed to Enquire into Certain Aspects of Opium and Ganja Consumption', *Assam Gazette*, 10 Dec. 1918, 1587.
[37] Ibid., 1583.

bhang when I had no money. We do not ordinarily smoke wild bhang because it causes headache and constipation.'[38] As such the Committee rather vaguely hoped for a cultural change rather than a state imposed prohibition. It pointed to 'village councils [that] if formed might do a good deal in the way of restricting the growth of wild bhang. The plant grows only in the neighbourhood of houses and it would not be difficult for an authority situated in the village to reduce it to a minimum.' In a similar vein the report urged 'that a Temperance Association should be organized to educate public opinion in Assam in connection with the use of intoxicants. As long as the demand for intoxicants exist, the stoppage or the excessive restriction of the illicit supply would only mean the substitution of an illicit supply.'[39] It seems that in Assam the colonial government was becoming increasingly aware of the limitations of its power in matters of drug consumption and was looking more and more to good intentions among the population as a means of checking the demand for cannabis.

Indeed, the picture from outside India and from elsewhere in the empire seems similar, in that the concern was to tax the trade in cannabis rather than to attempt to prohibit its use. The IHDC was confused as to whether the drug was banned in Trinidad but reports tended to suggest that a licence system existed there whereby the cultivator had to buy a permit to grow the crop. The expense of the permit had driven cultivation, which it was said had been extensive in the colony, into neighbouring Venezuela from where it was smuggled back into British territory.[40] However, twenty years later it seems that a new system had been introduced. The Ganja Ordinance of Trinidad 1915 established a system whereby all imported cannabis had to be stored in a Colonial Bonded Warehouse and collected only by traders that had paid a licence fee to the British authorities. In this the system came to resemble that operating in Bengal which was recommended by the IHDC. It seems that in the West Indies it was the government of British Guiana that had taken the initiative in updating mechanisms for controlling the ganja trade as it passed its Indian Hemp Ordinance in 1913.[41] Intriguingly, the laws in the West Indies were also instituted to control the habits of Indians. It is interesting to note that while many of the societies in the Caribbean are now popularly associated with

[38] Ibid., 1588.
[39] Ibid., 1586.
[40] 'The Policy of Hemp Drug Administration', in *Report of the Indian Hemp Drugs Commission*, i. 271.
[41] PRO HO 144/6073 29 Apr. 1924.

'ganja' consumption, the use of the plant for intoxicating purposes was first introduced there by Indians. They moved from Britain's territories in South Asia to the colonies as 'indentured labourers' throughout the nineteenth and twentieth centuries and took with them their favourite stimulant plant.[42]

EXPERIMENTS AND HALLUCINATIONS

While the IHDC report failed to have a major impact in British government and political circles cannabis itself was attracting rather more attention among medical and scientific groups in the period 1894 to 1912. Indeed, the interest in the drugs among those groups had continued sporadically throughout the last quarter of the century and cannabis medicines found themselves with a diverse range of advocates. In 1883 for example a debate on the medicinal uses of hemp preparations was sparked by the complaints of James Oliver, a doctor at the London Hospital for Women, about the uselessness of many of the hemp medicines that he had bought and of unpleasant effects of the drugs that had worked.[43] A 'Country Doctor' added that he had used cannabis medicines successfully to treat stomach and head aches but that his latest batch had produced unpleasant psychological side effects.[44] Further concern was expressed by John Brown, who wrote that 'in no case has it produced pleasurable feelings, generally most alarming symptoms such as complete paralysis, horrible hallucinations, double consciousness etc'. However he did admit that a preparation using tincture of cannabis indica had produced remarkable results in cases of menorrhagia and he was sure that the 'green medicine' might be considered the best way of treating the complaint.[45] Robert Batho wrote from the Isle of Man and was far more assertive about the benefits of cannabis medicines. He was confident that it was by far and away the best remedy for menorrhagia and indeed at no point in using it in his career in India were 'any disagreeable physiological effects observed'.[46] John Beddoe had used it to treat delirium tremens and was sure that none of his male patients had

[42] V. Rubin, 'The "Ganja-Vision" in Jamaica', in V. Rubin (ed.), *Cannabis and Culture* (Mouton Publishers, Paris, 1975).

[43] J. Oliver, 'On the Action of Cannabis Indica', *British Medical Journal* (Jan. to June 1883), 905.

[44] 'Cannabis Indica', ibid., 992.

[45] J. Brown, 'Cannabis Indica: A Valuable Remedy in Menorrhagia', ibid. 1002.

[46] R. Batho, 'Cannabis Indica', ibid. 1002.

[47] J. Beddoe, 'Cannabis Indica', ibid. 1064.

complained of 'disagreeable effects'[47] and Dr Cronin of Kensington was equally dismissive of these, insisting that cannabis prepared 'a most excellent nervine tonic'.[48] Further doctors wrote to attest to its power, including W. Peel Nesbitt from Adelaide in Australia.[49]

Finally, Surgeon Major Wallich, a friend and colleague of William O'Shaughnessy back in Calcutta in the 1830s, wrote to point out that he had used cannabis drugs to treat cholera, tetanus, and hydrophobia and that any differences in the experiences of the doctors was to be found in the source of their medicines. Only that produced from plants grown in tropical conditions could be guaranteed to be effective.[50] William Strange, the Senior Physician at the Worcester Infirmary, had more or less the final word on the subject in an article entitled 'Cannabis Indica as a Medicine and as a Poison' where he declared that excessive doses could indeed produce the 'disagreeable effects' of anaesthesia, mental confusion, and physical weakness. However, as a treatment for psychological problems he declared that he had always 'had a fondness for it' because of its good results.

A woman in acute melancholia said to me 'Doctor I must kill my children. Send me to an asylum'. I answered 'will you promise not to kill them until I have tried the effect of one medicine upon you?' She thought she could promise. A drachm of bromide of potassium, with half a drachm of tincture of cannabis, two or three times a day, in a fortnight caused so much improvement and even cheerfulness, that she declared she could now see the window open without the almost irresistible desire to throw her children down on to the pavement which had possession of her whole mind before.[51]

Occasional correspondence in the medical journals continued to recommend cannabis medicines to the British medical profession well into the 1890s. J. Russell Reynolds, Physician to the Royal Household, declared in 1890 that he had over thirty years of experience of the drug and that he was happy that 'Indian hemp when pure and administered carefully is one of the most valuable medicines we possess'. It was useful for calming those with insomnia, as a painkiller for wisdom teeth, for easing muscular spasms, and to relieve asthmatics. He was aware of the possible side effects and pointed out that both variations in the hemp plant and also in the tolerance of individuals to all vegetable based medicines accounted for the

[48] J. Cronin, 'Cannabis Indica', ibid. 1117.
[49] W. Peel Nesbitt, 'Cannabis Indica', ibid. 658.
[50] G. Wallich, 'Cannabis Indica', ibid. 1224.
[51] W. Strange, 'Cannabis Indica as a Medicine and as a Poison', *British Medical Journal* (July–Dec. 1883), 14.

sometimes adverse reactions to the drug. Responding to a letter in a previous edition of the *Lancet* that complained of 'an irresistible desire to commit suicide' after taking a dose of tincture of cannabis indica, Russell Reynolds simply pointed out that this would have been the result of the patient taking an excessive measure. As Russell Reynolds counted the Royal Household among his clients this letter is the origin of the myth that Queen Victoria was treated with cannabis. The correspondence at no point provides direct evidence for this.

The *Lancet* went on to report enthusiastically on French experiments with cannabis in gastric disorders and concluded that 'cannabis indica may be said to be a true sedative to the stomach'[52] while an American correspondent to the *BMJ* wrote advocating it in cases of migraine in 1897.[53] Caution about doses continued to be expressed in letters such as that from Antony Roche, who was Professor of Medical Jurisprudence and Public Health in Dublin. He warned of the perils of overdosing patients as he found one patient who had taken tincture of hemp in order to combat her migraine gripped by 'an inclination to jump down the stairs' and 'a creeping sensation in her arms and legs'.[54] However, his conclusion was related to the variable strengths of different tinctures rather than a call to abandon the mixtures altogether. Taken as a whole then this correspondence shows that in the last decades of the nineteenth century British doctors from all around the country and indeed from all around the empire were quietly and continually using medicines made from the hemp plant in the treatment of a wide range of complaints and ailments.

Indeed, where overtly negative reports of cannabis preparations entered the medical journals in this period it was not as comment on their efficacy as treatments but because of damning associations in India between the drugs and the lifestyles of those that used them as narcotics.

POISONING BY INDIAN HEMP: AUTOPSY.

The *Indian Medical Gazette* reports a case of death resulting from Indian hemp, some preparation of which the deceased had been accustomed to smoke for many years. After so indulging he generally became insensible or stupid. He was delirious for a fortnight before his death. On the day on which he died he tried to hammer a nail into his temple, and then expired suddenly... beneath the dura mater blood was found effused over the whole upper surface of right brain and

[52] 'Cannabis Indica in Gastric Disorders', *Lancet*, 2 (1890), 632.

[53] A. Stirling, 'Indian Hemp', *British Medical Journal*, 2 (1897), 691.

[54] A. Roche, 'Symptoms of Poisoning from a Small Dose of Tincture of Cannabis Indica', *Lancet*, 2 (1898), 1701.

over the frontal lobe of left brain. A large clot was found in the right middle fossa of skull; this extended across the crux and pons.[55]

However, both sides of the debates in India about the effects of hemp drugs in a society where they were regularly used as medicines and intoxicants were represented in the medical press. The *BMJ* for example recorded in 1894 that 'it is a significant circumstance, says the *Times of India*, that despite the outcry that has been raised as to the terrible effect of the consumption of hemp drugs, the lunatic asylums of the Central Provinces should have admitted only thirteen patients during this last year whose condition was attributable to this cause... those for which in the tables the smoking of ganja is assigned as the cause of admission form so small a proportion of the total number of lunatics as fairly to justify the elimination of all of these preparations from the lists of the causes inducing insanity'.[56]

Indeed, the Indian Hemp Drugs Commission merited a little attention in the medical journals of the period. The *Journal of Mental Science* had published a paper in January 1894 by Surgeon-Captain J. H. Tull-Walsh who was the Superintendent of the Lunatic Asylums in Calcutta and which was based on the evidence that he gave to the IHDC. His conclusions were tempered and rather more balanced that that of his predecessors discussed in Chapter 3. Ganja and bhang produced effects from mild exhilaration to marked intoxication in healthy individuals whereas among people with existing health problems even a moderate quantity acted to exacerbate the particular 'neuropathy'. 'Abuse of hemp drugs', which he did not clearly define, even in healthy persons could result in a condition resembling mania that could in time turn to melancholia and even to dementia. He felt however that in all cases absolute recovery could be depended upon and in those who did not recover after ten months there must already have been a pre-existing mental health problem.[57]

In a short reference to the IHDC report the *BMJ* summarized the reasons for the Commission in the first place. 'Hemp has been represented as a specially noxious substitute or alternative for opium in India. The use of haschish has been credited with terrible effects, violence, debauchery, insanity and crime. The gaols and madhouses of India have been said to be largely filled with its victims and rape and murder alleged to be frequently and directly due to excess in the smoking of ganja and drinking of bhang.' The *BMJ*, however, was careful to summarize the IHDC's refutation of

---

[55] 'Poisoning by Indian Hemp: Autopsy', *Lancet*, 2 (1880), 585.

[56] 'India and the Colonies', *British Medical Journal* (July–Dec. 1894), 108.

[57] J. H. Tull Walsh, 'Hemp Drugs and Insanity', *Journal of Mental Science*, 40 (1894), 36.

these charges: 'the report of the Hemp Drugs Commission has clearly demonstrated that this view of the effects of the consumption of hemp is grossly exaggerated, that the evils commonly attributed to its use do not exist and that the baneful effects caused by its abuse are very rare.'[58] Readers of the *BMJ* were reassured that 'it has been shown that in some parts of India the use of hemp in moderation is exceedingly common as many as 1 in 200 of the inhabitants of Bengal consuming it much as we in this country consume tobacco, tea or coffee or the inhabitants of France and Italy consume their cider or light wine'. The *Lancet* reported the conclusions rather more briefly:

As a result of the inquiry it appears that there are no such marked ill-effects, physical, mental, or moral, attendant on the use of hemp drugs as were popularly ascribed to them before the present inquiry was made. There was a complete breakdown in the evidence in support of the popular impression that these drugs are a fruitful source of insanity. There has, in fact, been a great deal of popular prejudice and exaggeration as to the evil effects arising from the use of hemp drugs and ganja.[59]

Indeed, it was in the *Lancet* that C. R. Marshall reported on 'The Active Principle of Indian Hemp' in 1897.[60] What this report revealed was that while doctors had been using cannabis drugs throughout the nineteenth century as a treatment for a variety of complaints, scientists had been working with the plant in order to try to isolate the active agent contained in cannabis. There seemed to be a direct link between the doctors and the scientists however as the notorious inconsistency in the quality of preparations complained of by the medical men had been the spur to researchers to try to locate the key ingredient in the plant. Marshall noted that 'the want of uniformity in the preparations of Indian hemp has so often led to serious consequences in practice that many practitioners have discarded the drug as worthless or dangerous. Others, finding it of benefit in certain diseases, have expressed a hope that some means of standardising it would be discovered or the active principle of the plant isolated.' His summary of scientific attempts to refine and further refine cannabis started with O'Shaughnessy, whom Marshall called 'the first European to investigate with any degree of scientific accuracy the action of Indian hemp'. In 1839 he had used alcohol as the purifying agent and had boiled freshly prepared ganja with spirit in his Papin's digester and had evaporated the spiritous extract so that a solid brown lump of concentrated cannabis remained.

[58] 'The Indian Hemp Drugs Commission', *British Medical Journal* (Jan.–June 1895), 938.
[59] 'The Hemp Drugs Commission', *Lancet*, 1 (1895), 1080.
[60] C. Marshall, 'The Active Principle of Indian Hemp: A Preliminary Investigation', *Lancet*, 1 (1897), 235–8.

After this initial effort, attempts to come up with pure extracts of active ingredients from samples of hemp preparations became rather more complicated. In 1846 T. and H. Smith tried digesting ganja in successive quantities of warm water until nothing was dissolving in the water, then they immersed what was left in sodium carbonate solution for two days over a moderate heat. The residue after all of this was extracted with rectified spirit and what remained was treated with milk of lime, which was filtered and the excess lime removed with sulphuric acid. A pinch of charcoal was put into the mixture and this was filtered. The final mixture was put back into water, which was allowed to evaporate and the solids were washed until free from acidity and bitterness. What they were left with was a resin, about 6 per cent of the original mass, which was potent indeed as 'two-thirds of a grain produced narcosis and one grain decided intoxication'. They named the resin cannabin.

Attempts to obtain resins that were purer still and that could be said to be the active ingredient of cannabis were made throughout the century both in Britain and across Europe. The Frenchman Personne published his results in 1857 and by distilling hemp in water he obtained an oily substance that contained two distinct compounds cannabebe ($C_{18}H_{20}$) and hydride of cannabene (C_6H_{14}). However, these substances did not seem to have the characteristic effects of cannabis drugs so it seemed unlikely that Personne had isolated the active ingredient. Indeed the Italians Vignola and Valenti conducted further experiments on the Frenchman's cannabene that showed that it was impure. The Russian Preobraschensky revealed that he had isolated nicotine from a hemp sample in 1876, but the Germans Dragendorff and Marquiss pointed out that this could be explained by the fact that he had been using a preparation of cannabis mixed with tobacco. The focus in the 1880s was on producing an alkaloid that contained the active ingredient and Siebold and Bradbury isolated a varnish-like base that gave alkaloidal reactions that they named cannabinine of which they managed to create two grains from ten pounds of the drug. Hay managed to isolate an alkaloid that apparently produced tetanus in frogs but not in cats. The Italians Zuco and Vignola also came up with an alkaloid which, unfortunately, failed to have the effects of cannabis drugs and so could not have contained the active ingredient.

Indeed, it was the British scientists Wood, Spivey, and Easterfield who, working with samples from India,[61] thought that they had finally succeeded

---

[61] C. Marshall, 'A Review of Recent Work on Cannabis Indica', *Pharmaceutical Journal*, 15 (1902), 132.

in obtaining what seemed to be a resin that was the active ingredient of cannabis. This was 'a toxic red oil or resin ($C_{18}H_{24}O_2$) boiling at 265 degC under a pressure of 20 mmHg yield 33 per cent'. Their success was in deriving the same substance from various forms of cannabis—from the Smiths' cannabine, from cannabis resin, from charas, and so on—and the authors decided to call their discovery cannabinol. They forwarded cannabinol to C. R. Marshall as he was the Assistant to the Downing Professor of Medicine at the University of Cambridge and as such was the man to conduct pharmacological trials of the substance. No doubt in the name of science, and with an admirable commitment to the cause, Marshall decided that there was no time to waste and that it was important to establish that cannabinol was active. One quiet afternoon when there was little going on and he was 'engaged in putting up an apparatus for the distillation of zinc ethyl', he popped about 0.1 gramme of cannabinol in his mouth and had a good suck on it while it dissolved. He found that it was slightly bitter and aromatic and that after a while it had a slightly anaesthetic effect on his tongue. The boredom of the afternoon pressed on and he settled himself to watch the zinc ethyl distilling away in the pharmacologist's equivalent of watching a kettle boil.

Forty-five minutes later he was wandering aimlessly around the room, failing to combat the urge to giggle, and repeating to himself the conclusion that 'this is lovely'. Suddenly, the apparatus that was distilling the zinc ethyl began to leak air and panic set in at the laboratory as the result of this could have been an explosion in the equipment. Marshall apparently found this hilarious 'I sat down and laughed incessantly for several minutes' and it was only because the drug had not fully taken a hold that he could be persuaded to help prevent a disaster. However, once the cannabinol was entirely in his system he found himself utterly intoxicated.

At one time, although walking rapidly, I felt cold and had to adjourn to an adjoining room where a fire was burning. I stood before it and thought how strange things were. I had a hazy notion of having been rational once and I wondered if ever I should be rational again. I was devoid of feeling, fearless of death, and even insensible to the feeling of others: if the friend by my side had died I think I should have laughed.

He was sent home by a doctor that had been called out by his anxious colleagues but after a couple of cups of coffee and a good dinner he felt entirely normal and went to a sound night's sleep. On a second occasion when he took the drugs, however, it took four hours for the effects to come on. He settled into a comfortable chair after lunch having taken 0.05

gramme ($\frac{4}{5}$ grain) at 2.35 p.m. and in no time 'a dreamy state supervened and visions of a grotesque character appeared. A regiment of soldiers was seen marching; their movements gradually increased to running, their legs went faster and faster, until finally the whole regiment was lost in a number of rapidly revolving circles. Then visions of ugly boys were seen; from slight ugliness greater ugliness developed, and this increased so as to become ridiculous.' At 9 p.m. he took himself off to bed. Indeed, such was the interest in the drug that he agreed to supply it to a friend who was suffering from insomnia. The treatment was a success and the patient slept soundly from midnight to 8 a.m., but not before he had been disturbed by similar hallucinations, 'one that I remember was a bow-legged boy running with a chest of tea between his legs; another seemed like a procession of females in the distance but on closer examination turned out to be coffins; these quickly melted away leaving nothing but confusion.'

Marshall was cautious in his conclusions about the possibilities of canna-bis as a medical substance: 'considerable experience is always needed to establish the usefulness of any medicine and this I have not yet been able to obtain,' he warned, though he did mention that cannabinol had been successfully used in cases where a hypnotic was required. W. E. Dixon, however, was far more confident in his assertions. He was the Salters's Research Fellow in Pharmacology and was based at St Thomas's Hospital in London. Professor Dunstan at the Scientific Laboratories of the Imperial Institute had taken up the work of Wood, Spivey, and Easterfield and he sent Dixon samples of the cannabinol that he had made together with samples of crude Indian hemp. Dogs, cats, and men were the subjects of Dixon's experiments and he was enthusiastic in his conclusions once he had tempered them with a warning about the problems of varying strengths of different preparations and the need to be able to isolate the active ingredi-ent.

I can affirm that it is soothing and stimulating when inhaled, being a specially valuable cerebral stimulant. I believe it to be an exceedingly useful therapeutic agent, one not likely to lead to abuse and producing in proper dosage no untoward after-effects ... the nervous effects produced may be such as to cause serious alarm, yet no danger is to be apprehended whilst the heart remains regular and strong.[62]

It seems that interest in the chemistry of cannabis continued into the twentieth century despite an incident of a tragic nature when one of the original trio of Cambridge scientists, Spivey, died during experiments with

[62] W. E. Dixon, 'The Pharmacology of Cannabis Indica', *British Medical Journal*, 2 (1899), 1356.

oxy-cannabin.[63] C. R. Marshall went on from his personal experiments with the drug in Cambridge to become Professor of Materia Medica and Therapeutics at St Andrews University in Scotland and to continue to work with cannabis. In 1903 he published a paper that confirmed his belief that the cannabinol of Easterfield, Spivey, and Wood was the active principle of Indian hemp and showed that while this substance could be broken down further its constituents when taken separately had no power to intoxicate. In 1911 he demonstrated that iodine and acetyl, which had been suggested as indicator tests for the potency of cannabis specimens, were poor means of examining the drugs and he disinterred a sample of the original cannabinol produced in 1897 to prove his point.[64] By this time, however, cannabinol was no longer considered to be the 'active ingredient' as Wood and Spivey had dismissed their own creation in 1898 at a meeting of the Chemical Society.[65] The search for an accurate test of the intoxicating power of cannabis was a response to the unsatisfactory way of establishing the potency of individual samples that was used at the time by drugs companies. This seemed simply to involve feeding a morsel of each batch to a group of dogs and seeing how long it took them to fall asleep.

An article in the *Edinburgh Medical Journal* of 1900 however points to the interest of another group in cannabis drugs. James Foulis had been called to the house of two brothers, one 'a medical student in his third year' and the other 'an art student, quite a philosopher in his way, and of a highly strung and sensitive nature'.[66] The former of the two admitted that 'with a view to experiencing the wonderful dreams said to be produced by haschish or cannabis indica my brother and I on three successive occasions took doses of that drug'. On the third occasion each took over 90 minims together with tablets that contained morphine. Both experienced sensory distortion, elation and depression and then hallucinations. One of the brothers wrote

It now dawned upon me that perhaps this escapade was going to end in death, and a most vivid picture presented itself to my mind. It was a picture showing Virgil and Dante standing on a rocky ridge overhanging a deep abyss, whence are issuing multitudes of lost souls on their way to Hades. I imagined myself standing on that ridge watching the unending and evermoving throng passing out of sight. Above me there seemed to be an irresistible force, dragging me most unwillingly

    [63] C. Marshall, 'A Review', 131.

    [64] C. Marshall, 'Report on the Standardization of Preparations of Indian Hemp', *British Medical Journal*, 1 (1911), 1171; *British Medical Journal*, 1 (1912), 1234.

    [65] 'Cannabinol', *Pharmaceutical Journal*, 7 (1898–9), 15.

    [66] J. Foulis, 'Two Cases of Poisoning by Cannabis Indica', *Edinburgh Medical Journal*, 8 (1900), 201.

from that spot. I told the doctor that I felt in the presence of death—that feeling described by patients who suffer from angina pectoris. The doctor assured me that the drug seldom proved fatal. This annoyed me extremely.

While medical experiments with cannabis flourished in Britain in the period 1894 to 1912 it seems that this was also a period when there was a growing interest in the country in the 'philosophical' possibilities of the plant's consciousness altering properties. Indeed, the medical and the intellectual were often closely related, in the above account it is a medical trainee and his artistic brother that try out the drug, and it is interesting to note that C. R. Marshall's own reports of the effects of doses of the drug on his mental state in 1897 were first reported to the Cambridge Philosophical Society before being written up for the *Lancet*. Indeed, some of the most important and creative literary figures of the 1890s incorporated cannabis substances into their lifestyles. When *Abkari* mentioned 'a club founded in London for hashish smoking'[67] in 1896 it was probably referring to the Rhymers Club. This was a loosely organized band of poets 'rebels in their art, opposed to Victorian morality, striving for sensibility rather than conscience, in love with beauty for its own sake'[68] that included W. B. Yeats and Ernest Dowson. They experimented with drugs such as opium and with other sensory stimulants including absinthe in order to enhance their creativity.[69] Yeats, who asked in his *Autobiographies* 'was modern civilization a conspiracy of the sub-conscious?'[70] wrote while in Paris that 'I take hashish with some followers of the eighteenth century mystic Saint Martin'.[71] John Addington Symonds described an afternoon with Dowson and a fellow member of the Rhymers Club, Arthur Symons,

Later on we tried the effect of hashish—that slow intoxication, that elaborate experiment in visionary sensations, which to Dowson at Oxford had been his favourite form of intoxication, which however had no effect on him as he sat, a little anxiously, with as his habit was, his chin on his breast, awaiting the magic.[72]

Related to the activities of these literary types was that of the occultists of the late nineteenth century. Maud Gonne, a girlfriend of Yeats's and an activist in Anglo-Irish political and mystical fringe groups in the 1880s and

[67] 'Hemp Drugs in North Africa', *Abkari*, 26 (1896), 100.
[68] N. Cardozo, *Lucky Eyes and a High Heart: The Life of Maud Gonne* (Bobbs Merrill, New York, 1978), 104.
[69] See J. Gardner, *Yeats and the Rhymers' Club* (Lang, New York, 1989), 173.
[70] W. B. Yeats, *Autobiographies* (Macmillan, London, 1926), 327.
[71] Ibid. 428.
[72] John Addington Symonds quoted in V. Berridge, 'The Origins of the English Drug "Scene" 1890–1930', *Medical History*, 32 (1988), 54.

1890s, discovered cannabis medicines as a cure for her insomnia and as a means of aiding her 'astral travel'. She claimed that under their influence she was visited by a shadow that told her 'you can now go out of your body and go anywhere you like, but you must always keep the thought of your body as a thread by which to return'.[73] Aleister Crowley adopted the nickname Great Beast 666 and eventually became regarded as 'the most dominant personality in occult circles at this period'. He began to try drugs as a student at Cambridge before heading to Mexico, India, and Egypt to sample the local narcotics and to develop a relationship with 'Aiwass', his guardian angel. He declared in 1920 that 'the action of hashish is as varied as life itself and seems to be determined almost entirely by the will or mood of the assassin and that within the hedges of his mental and moral form. I can get fantastic visions, or power of various kinds, or ravenous hunger, or vigour of imagination, whichever I please, absolutely at will on a minute dose of the Parke Davis extract.'[74]

It is worth noting the elite status of those that were using cannabis substances for other than purely medical reasons, for instance one of the brothers that tried out hemp drugs worried that 'the servants were listening to us'.[75] Those that experimented with the drugs for their artistic and philosophical possibilities were isolated individuals or at the most tiny groups that moved in restricted and affluently leisured circles. There was certainly no widespread use of cannabis substances in Britain or indeed in Europe in this period. Indeed, after the flurry of concern about the issue in India in the 1890s, the government in Britain lost interest in hemp narcotics and those campaigners that had focused attention on them as part of the anti-opium drive diverted their energies elsewhere. In the two decades after the IHDC the British occupied themselves with cannabis either in India, where the trade in hemp drugs continued to be a handsome source of tax revenue for the colonial state, or from time to time in the laboratories and journals of the scientific and medical world. In the latter a sporadic debate meandered on about the possibilities of cannabis medicines and about the difficulties of isolating the active ingredient from hemp samples so that it could be used as the basis for manufacturing more reliable drugs.

However, the issue of cannabis drugs and medicines was soon to be raised again for officials and politicians in Britain and in the empire. This was once again to happen because of broader and more urgent concerns

[73] S. Levenson, *Maud Gonne* (Cassel, London, 1976), 85.

[74] Aleister Crowley quoted in P. Haining (ed.), *The Hashish Club: An Anthology of Drug Literature* (Owen, London, 1975), 251.

[75] Foulis, 'Two Cases of Poisoning', 206.

about opium substances. The series of opium conventions that began in 1912 at The Hague and through which the international system of drugs controls that exists today was to evolve, was to put cannabis back on the British political agenda.

7

'An allusion was made to hemp in the notes appended to the Hague Opium Convention': The League of Nations and British Legislation, 1912–1928

INTERNATIONAL DRUGS POLITICS 1909–1923

By 1925 the British parliament was presented with draft legislation relating to cannabis that regulated possession and supply and by 1928 this legislation had been approved and had become law. This was the first British law on cannabis and cannabis products and yet between 1912 and 1928 there was no significant change in the patterns of use of cannabis in British society or British medicine. It remained largely unknown as an intoxicant and was infrequently used in medical practice. It was not therefore developments in domestic drug consumption that had inspired these new restrictions. Rather, and this is the key to understanding the origins of these laws, it was the rise of drugs controls as an international issue that lay behind the new legislation on cannabis in this period, and more specifically it was the politics of the international drug trade that meant that Indian hemp substances became the subject of statutory regulation.

The politics of the international drug trade might be roughly summarized as follows. Britain had made massive profits from supplying opium to China from India throughout the nineteenth century despite frequent attempts by the Chinese to control consumption by its population. They did not simply face British determination to sell the drug in trying to do this but also the resolve of China's suppliers who produced opium for the home market. However, by 1907 the British had unilaterally signed a treaty with the Qing Emperor that stated that they would reduce their exports to China over the next ten years by 10 per cent annually if the Chinese similarly reduced their production at the same rate. The net result, over ten years, would be the end of opium supply to the country. While there was initial scepticism over the Chinese commitment it seemed that they were indeed capable of sticking to their objectives so the British accelerated their pro- gramme and ceased exporting opium to China by 1913. They did continue supplying opium from India to British colonies throughout Asia such as Singapore and Hong Kong, where many Chinese nationals continued to buy the drug, often to smuggle back into China. Indeed, after 1911 the central government of China collapsed and the country once again slipped into producing opium for its domestic market, to much condemnation from the British and other international groups.

The British also continued to supply the Indian domestic market for opium where the drug was used as a medicine and as a tonic as well as a source of intoxication. Colonial rule in India also meant that the British controlled the world's largest producer of and market for cannabis products and, as seen in previous chapters, they levied duties on the drug there. These were raised with the avowed intention of limiting use by increasing the expense of cannabis products but this also conveniently brought in significant revenues for the administrations of India.

America had gained colonies in the Philippines at the end of the Span- ish-American war and had extensive trading interests with China. In the Philippines it inherited a population much taken to the consumption of opium and it also saw in its dealings with China the problems of a state beset by opium use in its subject population. Eager to trade with a strong China and keen to show itself to be an 'enlightened' colonial ruler in the Philippines the United States adopted a strident anti-opium stance. It took the initiative to organize an international conference on the issue in the first decade of the twentieth century and in 1906 began contacting a number of governments involved in the drugs trade. This culminated in the 1909 Shanghai Opium Commission from which was to grow the system of international regulation of all manner of drugs that continues to this day. The Americans remained firmly rooted to the simple idea that controlling drug use in a population was only a matter of cutting off the supply, preferably by curtailing agricultural production of the raw materials for processed drugs.

The 1909 Commission was heralded by Theodore Roosevelt as 'a fine example of what is best in modern civilization and international good-will and co-operation'.[1] In hindsight it looks more like an American attempt to set an agenda on international drug trading as the British delegates at the meeting noted that 'in the first instance the United States' delegates alone had attended the commission with resolutions that had been already pre-pared'.[2] These were rejected by the conference, which was also attended by representatives from thirteen countries including China and Japan, Persia, France, and Germany. The British and the Americans drew up a set of compromise resolutions that all could agree on as these involved few com-mitments and plenty of diplomatic hot air. The Commission recognized the commendability of 'the gradual suppression of opium smoking', urged the 'duty of adopting reasonable measures to prevent smuggling of opium' and emphasized 'the grave importance of controlling the manufacture, sale and distribution of morphine'.[3]

The Shanghai Commission was swiftly followed up in 1912 by the first of a series of meetings on the issue of drugs that was hosted by the govern-ment of the Netherlands at The Hague. These meetings quickly demon-strated that international dealings on narcotics were to be anything but the shining examples of 'international good-will and co-operation' that Roose-velt had envisaged back in 1908. Germany, for example, was a key produ-cer and exporter of morphine, heroine, and cocaine by the first decade of the twentieth century. Its pharmaceutical industry was keen to use the meetings to protect the lucrative trade in these products from rivals in Switzerland, the Netherlands, Peru, and Bolivia. Turkey and Persia remained major opium producers and attended only to safeguard their interests.

Indian hemp drugs appeared on the international agenda for the first time at this meeting as they were introduced by the Italians. It seems that they had come up with the issue as a suitable item for discussion at the International Opium Conference only at the last moment and it was cer-tainly the case that the British delegates felt that they had been given little time to look properly at the question before attending; 'the suggestion for the inclusion of hemp drugs in the conference programme was not brought to the notice of HM Government till about a fortnight before the conference met'.[4] Indeed, the British delegates wrote as if this last minute decision to

---

[1] President USA to the Senate and House of Representatives, 11 May 1908 in *Correspondence Relative to the International Opium Commission at Shanghai 1909* (HMSO, London, 1909), 4.

[2] From C. Clementi Smith to Edward Grey, 8 Apr. 1909, ibid. 7.

[3] Ibid. 8.

[4] *Report of the British Delegates to the International Opium Conference Held at the Hague, December 1911–January 1912* (HMSO, London, 1912), 14.

include cannabis for discussion at the meeting had caught the Italians rather by surprise as well, as it seemed that 'the Italian delegation was not to present any specific proposal in regard to hemp drugs, but rather to leave it to the conference as a whole to take such measures in regard to these as it might deem expedient'. In other words the Italian delegation had brought up the subject but seemed to have little to say on it.

In fact, the Conference as a whole seemed rather nonplussed about cannabis. The Programme Committee that had to decide where to squeeze it into the agenda raised a series of objections to having to do so. First of all, stated its chairman Mr Cremer, the Conference lacked any statistics for getting to grips with the importance of cannabis in the international drugs trade and secondly it seemed that none of the delegates had instructions from their governments about how to deal with the issue. He reasoned that it might not even be part of the international drugs problem which had until then been focused on opium and opiates. He therefore suggested that it would be sufficient for the countries threatened by the abuse of hemp drugs to take internal measures against them. Finally, he noted, it was not easy to know what ought to be discussed as it was difficult to obtain a scientific definition of the preparations that would have to be dealt with. Overall then, the Italian attempt to have cannabis placed on the agenda of the international efforts to regulate harmful narcotic substances was given short shrift by the Opium Conference of 1912, although the diplomats did do their best to make it look as if the Italian suggestion had been dealt with properly. A resolution on the subject was hastily formulated: 'il est désirer que les Gouvernements participants étudient la question du chanvre indien au point de vue statistique et scientifique, dans le but de régler éventuellement par leur législation intérieure ou pour un accord intérnational, les abus de son emploi.' The British delegation noted, with some satisfaction, that 'this resolution was carried with an amendment proposed by us substituting for the word "éventuellement" the words "si la nécessité s'en fait sentir" '.[5] In other words the issue was largely ignored as the Conference swept it aside with kind words about participating governments going off and doing their own scientific and statistical inquiries into the issue with the

---

[5] Ibid. 'It is desired that the participating Governments study the question of Indian hemp from a statistical and scientific point of view, with the goal of possibly regulating by their domestic legislation or by international agreement, the abuses of its employment.' The British insisted that 'possibly' be replaced with 'if it is felt necessary' so that the resolution read, 'It is desired that the participating Governments study the question of Indian hemp from a statistical and scientific point of view, with the goal of regulating, if it is felt necessary, by their domestic legislation or by international agreement, the abuses of its employment.' Author's own translation.

possible goal at some unspecified time of formulating regulations if they
seemed necessary. However, no mention of cannabis made it into the International Opium Convention signed at The Hague on 23 January 1912.
This focused entirely on 'the gradual suppression of the abuse of opium,
morphine and cocaine' and committed the contracting countries to a range
of laws and regulations controlling the manufacture, sale, and use of those
drugs in their various forms.

Quite why the Italians should have raised the subject in the first place is
a matter of some speculation. McAllister, in his study of the politics of the
opium meetings of this period, suggests that Italy and Austria only sought
invitations to these events in order to maintain the appearance of being
'Great Powers' by turning up alongside those countries that were truly
important.[6] The Italian insistence on placing something on the agenda may
simply have been part of this strategy of drawing attention to Italy's presence
on the world stage. Indeed, the fact that cannabis was introduced at a rather
late stage in the drawing up of the issues for the meeting together with the
lack of real ideas on the topic presented by the Italian delegation certainly
seem to point to other reasons for the inclusion of Indian hemp on the
agenda than a genuine concern about preparations of the plant.

However, Taylor's study of American diplomatic correspondence on the
opium meetings suggests that the Italians pointed to 'the trade in Indian
hemp and hashish, for which Italian territory served as a collection and
storage centre for smuggling into other territories'[7] as a justification for
including the drug on the Conference agenda. Citing Taylor, McAllister
embellishes this and concludes that the Italian concern was derived from
the fact that it was 'experiencing difficulty curbing a long-established trade
in marijuana and hashish through its African possessions'.[8] Italy, because
of its geographical location, was to remain at the centre of drug running
around North Africa and the Mediterranean for years to come. Harry
D'Erlanger's account of smuggling in the 1930s, *The Last Plague of Egypt*,
devoted a whole chapter to showing how Italian shipping lines were at the
heart of opium and cannabis smuggling organized by Greek gangs and
provided the following example.

While it had to work with the greatest discretion and care in order not to arouse
suspicion, the Bureau was aware that when the SS Umbria arrived at Alexandria

[6] W. McAllister, *Drug Diplomacy in the Twentieth Century* (Routledge, London, 2000), 28.
[7] A. Taylor, *American Diplomacy and the Narcotics Traffic 1900–1939* (Duke University Press,
Durham, NC, 1969), 87.
[8] McAllister, *Drug Diplomacy*, 31.

on January 17th 1931, the hashish was on board in five travelling trunks bearing counterfeit Italian Consular seals. The agent on board was also able to inform the Bureau that the hashish weighed over half a ton and that the trunks were to be passed unopened through the customs, thanks to a consular request for diplomatic facilities. The request took the form of a letter on the official stationery of the Italian Consulate-General at Alexandria which bore genuine Consular seals and the forged signature of the Italian Consul Judge.[9]

Indeed, the Italian delegation at the League of Nations Opium Committee under the leadership of Senator Cavazzoni was to return to the issue of smuggling throughout the 1920s and 1930s. The 1912 reference to cannabis by the Italians may therefore have been more than simply a political gesture. It can be seen as an early example of their concerns over the issue of illegal drug movements from their territory that was to grow in subsequent decades.

However, on the international drugs conference circuit cannabis products settled back into obscurity for over a decade after 1912. Indeed, the international drugs circuit itself was temporarily suspended due to the First World War. It was, however, quickly revived at the end of hostilities. The Hague Opium Convention featured in the 1919 peace treaties that brought the First World War to a formal end. Article 295 of the treaty signed by Germany, Article 247 of that with Austria, and Article 147 of that with Bulgaria stipulated that 'those of the High Contracting Parties which have not yet signed, or which have signed but not yet ratified, the Opium Convention signed at the Hague on January 23rd 1912 agree to bring the said Convention into force'.[10] Indeed, the drugs conferences themselves were reconvened under the authority of the League of Nations in 1921.

The Advisory Committee on Traffic in Opium met on 2–5 May of that year for the first time. The Dutch hosts chaired the initial session and the British, French, and Portuguese made up the European contingent, with the UK taking an extra place on the Committee to represent India. Japan, China, and Siam also sent representatives. The remit of the Committee was 'to secure the fullest possible cooperation between the various countries in regard to the carrying out of the Opium Convention and to assist and advise the Council in dealing with any questions that may arise'.[11] The Committee gradually expanded in numbers, Germany and the Serb-Croat-Slovene State were invited on in 1922 for example, and it set about the task of gathering information and suggesting policy. However, discussion did

---

[9] H. D'Erlanger, *The Last Plague of Egypt* (Lovat Dickson & Thompson, London, 1936), 199.
[10] *Report of the Advisory Committee on Traffic in Opium 1921*, p. 19.
[11] Ibid. 1.

not return to the subject of cannabis and it seemed forgotten during the sessions of the Committee and of the joint meetings that it held with the Health Committee.

Indeed, it is hardly surprising that issues other than that of opium, morphine, and cocaine were not considered during this time given the passions generated by the topics that were under discussion. These began to boil over with the arrival in 1923 of American representatives at the Advisory Committee. They immediately lined themselves up against the British governments and accused them of poisoning China. Bishop Brent, one of the American delegation who had worked for many years in Asia and who was a veteran anti-drugs campaigner, went straight for the moral and indeed the rhetorical high ground on his first day. He declared, with complete sincerity, that 'the United States, with her many faults and errors, stands honestly and firmly for the might of right and the commonwealth of mankind'.[12] He conjured up startling moral decisions in asserting that 'drug addiction is not only a disease, but a disease far more terrible than that which attacks the body only. I would choose for myself, or for anyone I loved, malaria, or smallpox, or yellow fever which kill the body in preference to drug addiction, which kills both body and soul.' He called upon the beneficence of the West in creating images of the weakness of the East: 'China is sick from head to foot of her body politic. We must figure out how we can best help her in her weakness and abjure any temptation to make profit out of her misfortune.' Then he pointed the finger.

Turkey, Persia, and India were the three principal opium producing countries, he noted, but of these it seemed that it was the latter that Brent considered to be the most blameworthy. The reason for this was quite clear to him. Turkey and Persia produced fine drugs that could have legitimate medical purposes whereas 'India, with her low grade opium, does not pretend to provide the market with a medicinal product'. It was, in Brent's words, 'time . . . for action' and his fellow American delegate Stephen Porter made it clear what this action should be. The Committee must recommend to the Assembly of the League of Nations that it declare all non-medicinal and non-scientific use of opium to be an abuse and that it exercise control of the production of the drugs so that no surplus above and beyond the needs of medicine and science could be produced.

Of course it was to the delegation from the Government of India that heads would have turned after such a speech. Representatives of Persia and

---

[12] Minutes of the Fifth Session of the Advisory Committee on Traffic in Opium and Other Dangerous Drugs 25 May 1923, p. 13.

Turkey had wisely refused to participate. Opium use for other than strictly medical and scientific purposes was still legal, although hedged in by regulations, in India. Opium produced in India was still exported to British colonies in East Asia and these stood accused of acting as entrepôts for smuggling into China. Indeed, after the American speeches it was the Chinese delegate who piped up to proclaim their words 'inspiring in the fight of this evil of world-wide concern'[13] and other speakers joined in the chorus of accusations that the British administration in India was 'engaged in a traffic that could not be defended'.[14]

In response to this broadside John Campbell, the representative of the Government of India, seemed hesitant: 'if Bishop Brent had had some unpleasant things to say he had said them in the pleasantest possible manner,' he burbled before trying to share the blame with China in arguing that 'the consuming government had to control consumption [while] the producing government had to control production'.[15] He tried to explain with reference to the latter point that the Government of India did indeed share the Americans' concern and that the treaties that it had made with China on the opium question showed that it had acted within the limits reasonable in the complex circumstances in which it found itself. Finally however, and perhaps sensing that he was not winning over his audience, he turned to muttering about the dangers of the Committee overstepping its powers:

The League of Nations' present mandate in this matter was to supervise the execution of the Hague Convention and it followed therefore that this was also the mandate of the Advisory Committee. If it now adopted authoritatively an interpretation which would be disputed, not only by his own but by other Governments, then it seemed to him that the Committee would be acting inadvisedly and would be giving some show of colour to the criticism that the League was setting up as a Super-State and was attempting to draw into its own hands all the power it could.[16]

The attitude of the Americans had crystallized around a conviction that it was necessary to stop production of the drugs in order to stop consumption. The British administration in India, however, argued that little would be achieved by stopping production in their colony while there was still a demand for the drug in Asia as other regions would simply step in to meet any shortfall in supply caused by a decrease in Indian production. In other words, it disputed the simplistic notion of the Americans and this would set the two governments on opposite sides of the drugs debates for a long

[13] Ibid. 16.   [14] Ibid. 22.   [15] Ibid. 19.   [16] Ibid. 19–20.

time to come. The UK government itself publicly stayed out of the fight but its representative Malcolm Delevingne did argue that it was a moderation of demand rather than supply that was the plank of its policy: '[the British Government] looked for an effective diminution of the demand, and consequently of the supply of raw opium which the American Delegation was so earnest in desiring'.[17]

The Fifth Session of the Advisory Committee on Traffic in Opium and Other Dangerous Drugs broke up on 7 June 1923 with the final meetings still focusing on India, Persia, and Turkey as the key producers of opium. Campbell of the India Office still stoutly defended his government's position: 'the consuming countries were entirely free to consider what would be best in their own interests and the Government of India was ready to limit its exports to the certified requirements of the consuming countries,' he repeated three days before the end of the session. In other words he had not shifted from his original position adopted back in May, of reiterating that the British in India would continue to provide opium requested by other governments in order to satisfy the demands of their populations and that it would cease to supply opium to these countries only when they ceased to ask for it. To unilaterally cease the supply of opium would not end the consumption of the drug, it would simply encourage other producers to meet the demand, achieving nothing but a decrease in revenue in India.

By the end of the Fifth Session of the Advisory Committee in 1923 much heated debate had been generated but little progress had been made on the key issue of opium production. Cannabis meanwhile had been altogether forgotten by those so earnestly occupied by this issue. However, this was about to change. Towards the end of 1923 and while the Advisory Committee was in recess, a letter arrived in The Hague for the consideration of the group when it reconvened in 1924. It read as follows.

Pretoria November 28th 1923

With reference to your letter no. 12/A/22951/17217 dated September 6th 1922, on the above subject and to my letter no. 29/8/85 dated December last, forwarding copies of the Regulations promulgated under Proclamation no. 181 of 1922, I have the honour to inform you that, from the point of view of the Union of South Africa, the most important of all the habit-forming drugs is Indian hemp or 'Dagga' and this drug is not included in the International List. It is suggested that the various Governments being parties to the International Opium Convention should be asked to include in their lists of habit-forming drugs the following:

---

[17] Minutes of the Fifth Session of the Advisory Committee on Traffic in Opium and Other Dangerous Drugs 25 May 1923, p. 21.

Indian hemp: including the whole or any portion of the plants cannabis indica or cannabis sativa.

Signed, JC. Van Tyen, for Secretary to the Prime Minister.[18]

Cannabis was about to enter the deliberations of the Advisory Committee and was to become tangled, once again, in the politics of opium.

THE LEAGUE OF NATIONS AND CANNABIS

The Campbell/Delevingne Double Act

Straight after lunch on 12 August 1924, at the Twelfth Meeting of the Sixth Session of the Advisory Committee on Traffic in Opium and Other Dangerous Drugs, the British delegate Malcolm Delevingne and Campbell of the India Office made reference to the letter from South Africa in order to draw attention to the cannabis issue. It was Campbell who spoke first and he assured the Committee that the Government of India was already dealing with the issue. He told his colleagues that it had been informed of the South African communication and that it had acted promptly to consult the various administrations in India so as to discover whether it would be possible to prohibit the export of Indian hemp. He suggested leaving a full consideration of the subject for future sessions in order to allow time for information to be collected. Delevingne supported this suggestion and pointed out that the British government was also well ahead of others as it too had been collecting information on the subject of Indian hemp. Indeed, he even had a report to hand about the extent of the problem

---

[18] The letter confused 'dagga' with 'dakka' in the language of local drug users in South Africa. The former was the African word for the leaves of the *Leonotus* plants, which were smoked, the latter the local slang for cannabis preparations. The reason for the South African concern in the first place is explained by the labour politics of the region during the establishment of the colonial economy there. Indian migrants were sent from Asia to South Africa to work on the plantations there from the middle of the nineteenth century and seem to have taken the habit of using cannabis as a medicine and intoxicant with them. However, the white employers loathed anything that they feared would interfere with the docility and effectiveness of their workforce and it was complained that 'smoking of hemp . . . renders the Indian Immigrant unfit and unable to perform with satisfaction to the employer, that work for which he was specially brought to this Colony' (in *Report of the Indian Immigrants Commission (Natal Legislative Council) 1885–87* (Davis, Pietermaritzburg, 1887), 263). As it seems that the local African population also enjoyed cannabis preparations, the plant caused the colonial owners no end of anxiety (see B. M. du Toit, 'Dagga: The History and Ethnographic Setting of cannabis sativa in southern Africa' in V. Rubin (ed), *Cannabis and Culture* (Mouton Publishers, Paris, 1975), 81–116). Indeed, as early as 1870 the Governor of the Natal colony was given the power to make rules for controlling cannabis use.

that the British and the Government of India had made clear they were already doing so much to investigate.

Ten tons of this plant had recently been exported to Abyssinia, the owner of the consignment alleging that it was to be used as an insecticide. The consignment had reached the Port of Djibouti but eventually after a series of operations, it had disappeared entirely. Enquiries made by the British and French Governments left little room for doubt that it had been smuggled into Egypt for illicit purposes.[19]

This mention of the French government prompted its representative to get up and explain the policy of his country's colonies and he was adamant that when it came to cannabis 'he did not think that the time had yet to come to raise the question nor to suggest remedies'. The American delegate, Edwin Neville, seemed similarly unconcerned about the issue and asked pointedly if it was the case that any government had actually expressed a desire for the question to be discussed. Campbell was quick to reply, although not directly to his question, stating that 'the Government of India had taken up the question in advance from the point of view of prohibiting export should that appear desirable'. The Committee approved Malcolm Delevingne's proposal that governments should be asked to provide more information on Indian hemp and a questionnaire was circulated.

The issues of Indian hemp and the South African letter seem to have been brought up in a carefully coordinated manner by the British and India Office delegates, as both Delevingne and Campbell had their facts well marshalled and the positions of their respective governments well rehearsed. Why this should have been the case can be seen in the broader context of the day's discussions. Business on 12 August had been brisk indeed at the Committee. The morning of the 12th had seen wrangling over the Draft Agreement to be drawn up and presented to the forthcoming League of Nations Second Conference on Opium. Article 2 had been the source of some controversy as it stated that 'each Government undertakes to refuse to authorise the importation into its territory of any of the substances mentioned in Article 1 beyond the quantities specified in the estimates furnished by it in pursuance of Article 1'.[20] In other words here was a stipulation that very much focused on the consuming country and which was, therefore, in line with the Government of India's stance that consuming nations had as

---

[19] Minutes of the Sixth Session of the Advisory Committee on Traffic in Opium and Other Dangerous Drugs, 12 Aug. 1924, p. 52. The details of this smuggling case, which centred on the mariner Henri de Monfreid, can be found in PRO HO 144/6073 and is discussed again later in this chapter and at length in Chapter 8.

[20] Minutes of the Sixth Session of the Advisory Committee, p. 48.

great a role to play in addressing the international drug trade as did the producers. The Americans, of course, were rather more concerned to focus on the suppliers and their delegate made this point in relation to the above article as he made it clear 'it was in his opinion... the intention of the Committee to frame a scheme which would, in some degree, place responsibility upon the country of production and exportation'. However, he could not object to the idea of 'double responsibility', that is of both exporters and importers doing what they could to regulate the trade, so the article was passed. The session had very much gone to the advantage of the Government of India, with the ample assistance of the British delegation, as it had succeeded in shifting some of the emphasis on to consuming countries.

Indeed, the afternoon session faced a tough agenda that would once again pit the British and the India Office against the Americans. Some members of the Committee had sat with representatives from the League of Nations Health Committee on a Mixed Sub-Committee to consider the issue of setting quotas for each nation's requirements of each of the harmful drugs under discussion. It had submitted its conclusions, such as an estimate that each country needed 600 milligrammes of raw opium per head of population, and its recommendations were to be considered by that afternoon's meeting of the Committee on Traffic in Opium and Other Dangerous Drugs. Campbell of the India Office had sat on the Mixed Committee and had disagreed with its findings but it had ignored him and gone ahead and made its recommendations anyway. The British delegation also contested its report and Delevingne stated that while this concluded that heroin was unnecessary in medical practice and might therefore be completely prohibited this was certainly not the opinion of medical authorities in Britain. Campbell and Delevingne wanted the report of the Mixed Committee simply to be noted rather than to be recommended and also wanted the Opium Committee to withdraw its members from the Mixed Committee which would effectively close it down.

Neville, the American, naturally chose to oppose this. He ignored the poor treatment of Campbell on the Mixed Committee and instead chose to provide evidence for the report's conclusion that heroin was dispensable in medicine. He cited evidence from both military and public health services in the USA and told the Committee that heroin was not now considered important there and that indeed import of opium to manufacture it was now forbidden by Act of Congress. However, the British and Campbell of the India Office succeeded in their agenda and the Advisory Committee agreed simply to 'note' the report instead of endorsing its recommendations and to order that its members be withdrawn from future participation in the Mixed Committee.

The Campbell/Delevingne double act on cannabis might therefore be seen in the light of the day's business and indeed in the context of the rivalries that dominated the League of Nations' deliberations on drugs. It appeared after a session in which the British and British India delegations had had their way and had negotiated the insertion of an Article that very much bolstered the Government of India's strategy of focusing attention on opium consumers rather than solely on opium producers. It came just before the proposal by Campbell of the India Office, supported by Delevingne and the British, that the conclusions of the Mixed Committee should be given a lukewarm reception and indeed that its activities ought to be ended. The cannabis issue, when raised by the British and the India Office, gave both the opportunity to appear active and constructive on drugs issues on a day when they were otherwise pursuing their own well-defined agendas on the important issue of opium. By seeming to take seriously the issue of Indian hemp when others on the Committee gave the impression that they were not really interested in it, and also by revealing that their respective governments already had the matter in hand, Campbell and Delevingne were bolstering their position in the day's play. Having gained advantage in the morning, and with a tough afternoon's battling to be had, it served their purposes to focus on a drugs related topic just after lunch which was of little importance in the context of the larger debates about opium but which allowed them to demonstrate their concern over drugs issues by stating that it was being dealt with vigorously and effectively. No one on the Committee much cared about Indian hemp as they were there to discuss opium and cocaine and there was much controversy still to be had on those subjects. The British and the India Office therefore lavished attention on cannabis simply to gain a few minutes on the moral high ground to boost their position when it came to fighting in the opium trenches.

Indeed, in the context of the overall politics of the Conference, the selection of an issue that was of little concern in general but upon which the British and India Office delegations might appear forward thinking and active was a useful negotiating tool for Delevingne and Campbell. The Americans had arrived with radical proposals in 1923 and pursued these until their representatives walked out of the Second Opium Conference in 1925. The British had consistently stalled and obstructed them for a variety of reasons and Campbell was aware that the constant objections on his part were casting his role at the proceedings as that of reactionary and regressive.

The attitude of the Indian delegation was none the less misunderstood and was in some quarters characterised as obstructive. It was implied that India's reason for objecting to discussion was that the American proposal constituted an advance on the Hague Convention and that if it were once discussed, she could show no valid case against its adoption; perhaps, also, that she wished to conceal some failure to implement her existing obligations under the Hague Convention itself.[21]

The Indian hemp issue then was one that suited the British and the India Office tactics on 12 August 1924, but it was also useful for them in the broader currents of the League's drug meetings as it afforded them a rare opportunity to appear constructive. It was an issue that little concerned the other nations present—indeed the Americans had to ask why it was being mentioned at all—but it was one on which Delevingne and Campbell could appear to be pioneers of concern, a position that would promote their credentials as drug experts and campaigners that were otherwise disputed by those who felt that they were defending unhelpful positions on opium. In fact in order to appear progressive on Indian hemp they actually had to offer very little, simply pointing to inquiries that their governments had already made and suggesting that other interested countries might do the same. In short, the sudden British interest in cannabis in 1924 had little to do with the issue itself, and more to do with bargaining positions on opium.

The Egyptian and American Ambush

The matter might have met the same fate as the Italian interest in the same subject of 1912 had it not been for the Second Opium Conference that was assembled in 1924. While the Advisory Committee only invited delegates that claimed to have direct interests in the opium issue the Conference was open to representatives of all of the countries that were members of the League of Nations. It was assembled solely to meet two specific objectives. The first was to devise schemes to set maximum limits on the amounts of morphine, heroin, and cocaine that could be manufactured from raw opium and coca and also to restrict the production for export of the raw materials from which those drugs were made. The second was the amendment of the Hague Convention of 1912 so as to take account of the schemes devised to achieve the first objective.

However, from the outset it seemed that certain countries intended to use the meeting to air other grievances and to focus attention on other issues in the drugs debate. The United States, for example, made a proposal that

[21] International Opium Conferences at Geneva, 1924–25: Report of the Indian Delegation, in Maharashtra State Archives 1926 File 5639/24C, p. 3.

'the contracting parties shall enact effective laws or regulations for the control of the production and distribution of raw opium and coca leaves so that there will be no surplus available for purposes not strictly medical or scientific'.[22] Such a suggestion took the scope of the meeting way beyond the original subject of the Conference. The key objective of the international meetings to that date had been to ensure that the nations involved would agree not to supply the people of another country with opium or cocaine where the government of that country had banned or limited access to the drugs. It had urged countries to combat the demand of their peoples for the substances but had never attempted to force governments to impose regulations on their own peoples. The American motion implied an unprecedented intervention by the League of Nations to stamp its will on populations over and above the national sovereignty of their own governments. It would have meant that the League of Nations insisted that national governments enforce domestic policies that decreed that the only legitimate use of opium and coca drugs was 'medical' or 'scientific'. The focus would have shifted from regulating international trade between governments to forcing domestic policies on them. The Americans had already tried to put such a motion on the schedule of the Conference at the meetings of the Advisory Committee in 1923 that was setting the agenda for the Conference but they saw their proposal rejected there. As such they simply ambushed the proceedings of the Second Conference and it was the eventual rejection of this American proposal that caused them to storm out halfway through its proceedings.

Once the Americans had foisted their concerns onto the agenda regardless of what had already been agreed as the business of the meeting, other delegations similarly seem to have decided to press their own issues. Bishop Brent had stood and made the American proposal on the afternoon of the third day of the Conference in the afternoon. On the morning of the next day, as controversy bubbled about the nature of the American intervention, Dr Mohamed A. S. El Guindy, the head of the Egyptian delegation, stood to make his first contribution. The Chinese delegate had already praised the American agenda, and the Canadian and Romanian speakers did little more than wave at the diplomatic spotlight by issuing friendly hellos and assurances of cooperation on the parts of their governments without actually offering anything pertinent to the proceedings.

---

[22] International Opium Conferences at Geneva, 1924–25: Report of the Indian Delegation, in Maharashtra State Archives 1926 File 5639/24C, p. 5.

When El Guindy launched off on his speech the other delegates may well have shuffled their papers, as it had all the makings of a piece of empty diplomatic posturing much like the Canadian and Romanian efforts. 'I take this opportunity of offering this assembly, which includes so many distinguished men, the best wishes of my Government for the success of its work,' he waffled before continuing in a similar vein: 'conscious of her duty towards the whole human race, independent Egypt will do all that lies in her power to cooperate loyally and disinterestedly on the work which is before us'. Unexpectedly, however, he suddenly threw two suggestions at the other delegates:

The illicit use of opium and its derivatives and of the other substances mentioned in the Advisory Committee's report is universally condemned by public opinion. There is, however, another product which is at least as harmful as opium, if not more so, and which my Government would be glad to see included in the same category as the other narcotics already mentioned—I refer to hashish, the product of the cannabis indica or sativa. This substance and its derivatives work such havoc that the Egyptian Government has for a long time past prohibited their introduction into the country (except of course the trifling quantity required for medical purposes). I cannot sufficiently emphasise the importance of including this product in the list of narcotics the use of which is to be regarded by this Conference. I hope soon to be in a position to submit to this Conference a short memorandum on this question which is of such importance to my country.

It should be an accepted principle that all narcotic substances which are already known and which although not classed among injurious drugs may yet be regarded as such, together with all other narcotic products which may be discovered or produced in the future, should fall automatically within the scope of the measures of the Convention which we hope to conclude.[23]

He received applause for this ambitious speech, which at once suggested that a new drug be added to the scope of the Conference and indeed that the remit of every future agreement on drugs ought to be expanded to include all dangerous substances, even those that had yet to be discovered or created. The rest of the morning's session was dominated by a return to empty expressions of support for the Conference from countries such as Luxembourg and the Dominican Republic, to the considerable exasperation of the British delegate Malcolm Delevingne, who stood to complain that for all the previous few days' speeches he was still in the dark about the attitude of most of the delegates to the stated agenda of the Conference. He was one of the key movers behind the carefully limited agenda and was

---

[23] *Records of the Second Opium Conference*, vol. i, 20 Nov. 1924, pp. 39–40.

keen to ensure that it was observed. Ignoring Delevingne's interjection, the Turkish delegate took the Conference right back off that agenda again, arguing that 'there is in the case of Turkey another question, namely, that of hashish. There are special laws in Turkey to prevent the cultivation of, and trade in, hashish.' Clearly, the spirited hijacking of the agenda by a variety of groups was to be a permanent feature of the meetings.

By Saturday Delevingne was still trying to limit the Conference to the official agenda. He stood and made a speech that reminded the delegates that their objective was solely to consider measures for regulating the international trade in opium and cocaine drugs. For all the debates of the last few days about what was and was not to be discussed at the Conference, it was this issue alone, he maintained, that had been agreed as the remit of the gathering. Dr El Guindy rose immediately to do his best to divert the Conference from the agenda carefully stipulated by the British representative. 'I think that before beginning our work, it would be advisable to make an addition to the list of drugs. "Hashish" is not mentioned and I think it essential that it should be included.'[24] His Greek colleague Mr Dendramis stood up to support El Guindy's proposal and he also endorsed the other point made during the Egyptian's first speech that 'it would be better therefore if the word drug were taken to mean any harmful drug already known or which may be discovered'. Spotting another ambush of the agenda, Stephen Porter of the United States delegation seized the moment and made his attack, pointing out that he would find it difficult to stay at the Conference if the American suggestions made a couple of days earlier were not to be discussed at the gathering. The Egyptians and Americans combined to steer the Conference off the narrowly defined agenda that had been originally set out for it and to which Delevingne and the British phalanx were trying to keep it.

Delevingne was polite about El Guindy's interjection. It was 'a very interesting proposal', he decided, but it was already in hand. He explained that the Advisory Committee had previously organized a survey of the subject and had sent out questionnaires to the League's governments in order to gather information. He revealed that, alas, this had only happened in November 1924[25] and so the results had yet to arrive. He assured El Guindy that when the questionnaires were returned they would be

---

[24] *Records of the Second Opium Conference*, vol. i, 22 Nov. 1924, pp. 47.

[25] The questionaire was in fact only dispatched on 17 November 1924. The South African proposal had been discussed as long ago as 12 August by Campbell and Delevingne and the motion authorizing the questionnaire had been passed on 29 August. See See PRO HO 144/6073 Traffic in Indian Hemp 24 Nov. 1924.

looked at by the Advisory Committee. Until then, El Guindy was free to supply the Conference with all the information that he had and this would be forwarded to the Advisory Committee which, Delevingne assured him, would consider it at its meetings next year. He then turned to dealing with the American attempt to hijack the agenda and suggested that this be relegated to a matter for the consideration of subsidiary Committees instead of the Council itself. The delegates listened patiently to this and then headed for lunch.

As soon as the meeting to examine Delevingne's agenda was reconvened at 3.30 p.m. up stood the Egyptian as the first speaker, to make his two points once again. He promised to submit a formal proposal to include 'hashish' on the agenda and also one that advanced his opinion that 'we ought not to regulate the use of opium and its derivatives only but of all noxious drugs'.[26] He also took Delevingne to task about his attempt to delay discussion of cannabis until some indefinite point in the future: 'am I to understand by this that if, after reading the short statement I am preparing upon this question, the majority of the delegates of the Governments represented at this Conference were in favour of my proposal, it would nevertheless be impossible for us to take a decision in the matter at this Conference?' It was obvious that El Guindy, unlike the Italians and the South Africans that had half-heartedly raised the issue of cannabis at the international level in the past, was not going to allow the topic to be sidelined or delayed. Indeed, on this occasion the Turkish delegate stood and gave again his full support to his Egyptian colleague: 'during the general discussion I alluded to another scourge in addition to opium from which certain countries suffer. The proposal of the Egyptian delegate makes provision for this.'[27] The president of the Committee intervened to move the meeting on. He insisted that El Guindy should get on with it and submit a formal proposal if he intended to do so. Delevingne did not return to the subject that day.

El Guindy did indeed get on with submitting his official proposal and on the afternoon of 13 December he stood to make his bid to have hashish, which he described as the resin of the flowers, leaves, or hairs of the cannabis sativa plant, included on the list of narcotics with which the Conference had to deal. He rose to the occasion. 'Hashish is a toxic substance, a poison against which no effective antidote is known,' he declared and he outlined the effects of the drugs on human behaviour:

[26] *Records of the Second Opium Conference*, vol. i, 22 Nov. 1924, p. 55.
[27] Ibid. 56.

Taken in small doses, hashish at first produces an agreeable inebriation, a sensation of well being and a desire to smile; the mind is stimulated. A slightly stronger dose brings a feeling of oppression and of discomfort. There follows a kind of hilarious and noisy delirium in persons of a cheerful disposition, but the delirium takes a violent form in persons of a violent character. It should be noted that behaviour under the influence of the delirium is always related to the character of the individual. This state of inebriation or delirium is followed by a slumber, which is usually peaceful but sometimes broken by nightmares. The awakening is not unpleasant; there is a slight feeling of fatigue but it soon passes.

Larger doses were likely to have more dramatic results. El Guindy described 'a furious delirium and strong physical agitation; it predisposes to acts of violence and produces a characteristic strident laugh. This condition is followed by a veritable stupor which cannot be called sleep. Great fatigue is felt on awakening and the feeling of depression may last several days.' In short, he was saying that if the user overdid it, he would become insensible and suffer a hangover.

The chronic user, that is the regular and habitual consumer of 'hashish', suffered other problems. There was an impact on his physical frame as 'the whole organism decays' and on his mental health as 'the addict very frequently becomes neurasthenic and eventually insane'. This latter point was one that he returned to later in the speech as he stated boldly that 'illicit use of hashish is the principal cause of most of the cases of insanity occurring in Egypt ... generally speaking, the proportion of cases of insanity caused by the use of hashish varies from 30 to 60 percent of the total number occurring in Egypt'. Indeed, cannabis use did not simply lead to insanity, it was the first step on the slippery slope of drug abuse that meant that users would find themselves attracted to 'virulent poisons which they would never have dreamed of taking' before their first experiments with hashish. Here was the accusation that cannabis was not simply an evil in itself but that it was a gateway to the use of other dangerous drugs.

El Guindy had described the problems. Then he pointed to the solution. 'As early as 1860, Dr Mohammed Ali Bey made a report to the competent authorities regarding the accidents caused by the abuse of hashish. In 1884 the cultivation of this plant was forbidden. The cafes (or mashhashas) in which hashish was consumed by smoking in special hookahs were closed and are still mercilessly sought out by the police.' In 1924 the Egyptian customs service alone had seized 3,262,227 kg of hashish, so it was clear that the demand for the drugs was being met by illegal supplies from abroad. It was here that the Egyptians saw the need for international help. Including hemp narcotics in the international regulations drawn up at this Conference by the League of Nations would act to enlist the aid of other governments in controlling their exports of the drug, which would add another obstacle to the movement of hemp narcotics to markets in Egypt.

Demonstrating an awareness that most of the countries present would not have experience of cannabis users in their populations and as such would not have a direct interest in accepting his proposal to include cannabis on the League of Nations list of proscribed drugs, he issued a couple of dark threats to them. If hashish was not included on the list while opium and cocaine were, then he was sure that the drug that he was discussing would replace them and 'become a terrible menace to the whole world'. He wanted the other countries to act now to prevent the spread of this cannabis curse, or else, he warned, they would soon be meeting in order to cure it. Moreover, if they did not act now then the League of Nations itself would be undermined, 'for I know the mentality of Oriental peoples and I am afraid that it will be said that the question was not dealt with because it did not affect the safety of Europeans'.

In the half-hour of the speech he conjured up images of a horrific problem, he had other countries sympathize with the plight of his own, he assured them that his own government had acted energetically, he pointed to the international crime of smuggling, and he warned them that their own countries faced this scourge and that the prestige of the League of Nations itself was at stake. His performance, rounded off by this dramatic last paragraph, received prolonged applause.

I am certain that you gentlemen who work under the aegis of the League of Nations, will help us in the struggle we have undertaken against this scourge which reduces man to the level of the brute and deprives him of health and reason, self-control and honour.[28]

The Conference seemed stunned by his oration. The Chinese delegate stood and announced, 'I am greatly moved by the statement made by the honourable delegate of Egypt. While I know next to nothing about the subject ... I wish to assure the Egyptian delegate that it can count on us to do all we can to support its efforts.' He received applause for this. Next, the American stood and, apparently in all seriousness, declared that 'by helping each other we can made the world much happier and much better'. The delirium continued as this also drew applause. The British delegate for India, Mr Clayton, rose and summoning the full power of the

---

[28] All quotes from *Records of the Second Opium Conference*, vol. i, 12 Dec. 1924, pp. 132–5.

professional bureaucrat, delivered a spectacularly sobering slap to the proceedings: 'in my view, the administrative obstacles in the way of including any specific article dealing with hashish are, under the circumstances, extraordinarily great'. Unsurprisingly, this failed to get a clap, as did Sir Malcolm Delevingne's reminder that 'there are however, difficulties in the way of dealing with the matter here and now'. The British had spoiled the fun and insisted that hashish remained off the official agenda. Delevingne suggested that 'it might be possible for the interested Powers to continue the conversations which have already been begun in private, to exchange their views and information and experiences, and to arrive at an understanding so far as possible as to the measures that are desirable and the points on which it may be necessary to obtain further information. Personally, I should have no objection at all to the appointment of a small committee for continuing that work.' The 'interested Powers' that he alluded to were France and British India, so he was effectively suggesting that El Guindy be closeted away with representatives of the two nations that had between them tried to rule Egypt as an imperial possession for the best part of the previous 100 years.

The last thing that El Guindy wanted was to have the issue relegated to a small committee on which he would be outnumbered by the former colonial oppressors of his country. As such he made a final stab at forcing to a vote there and then his proposal that the resin of cannabis sativa ought to be included on the schedule of drugs: 'my main point was that hashish ought to be included in the list of narcotics since it has been recognised as such by all the members of the conference'. The president of the Committee would not allow such a vote and asked instead if he wanted to accept Delevingne's proposal or the American alternative. Stephen Porter of the US delegation had offered El Guindy a lifeline as he had suggested that hashish be referred to Sub-Committee F. This had been appointed to look at the issue of drugs other than raw opium such as heroin and cocaine. This was to be a fully international board rather than the French/British alliance proposed by Delevingne and would have the right to report back to the full Conference, which would once more give El Guindy the opportunity to grab its attention. He accepted the American proposal and the issue of cannabis was sent to Sub-Committee F for review. It seems that the Egyptians and the Americans, as the two chief hijackers of the agenda, were helping each other out and indeed in the context of the day's proceedings this seems even more obvious. Only that morning, El Guindy had addressed the Conference on the controversial American proposals on opium and had declared that 'I can only express my admiration for the purposes of those who desire to save the victims of this horrible drug in every country of the world. I most heartily support the American proposal.'[29]

Egypt and Sub-Committee F

El Guindy's speech made it clear that he had been lobbying extensively before he gave his address. He thanked the United States, Turkey, Japan, Brazil, Poland, and Greece for their promises of support. He also mentioned that he had had a meeting with the delegates of France, India, and Britain but that they had been unable to agree with El Guindy's demand for an immediate application of the Hague Opium Convention to cannabis. It seems then that he had his allies and his opponents well defined by the time he went to Sub-Committee F.

As such it came as no surprise to see the Greek, Brazilian, American, Japanese, and Turkish representatives on Sub-Committee F all stand to make various declarations on the evil of cannabis and the need for its inclusion on the Convention. The British delegate Mr Perrins did little more than ask for an exact definition of the term 'hashish' and the first meeting on the subject of cannabis was dissolved as the French, the India Office, the Egyptian, and the Turkish delegates were appointed to prepare a text for the consideration of the Sub-Committee. The result of this group was paragraph 6 of Sub-Committee F's recommendations for the full Conference that read as follows.

The use of Indian hemp and the preparations derived therefrom may only be authorised for medical and scientific purposes. The raw resin (charas) however, which is extracted from the female tops of the cannabis sativa together with the various preparations (hashish, chira, esrar, diamba etc.) of which it forms the basis, not being at present utilised for medical purposes, in the same manner as other narcotics, may not be produced, sold, traded in etc. under any circumstances whatsoever.[30]

It seems that there was little general interest in the issue of cannabis and that the Egyptian delegate had therefore been able to have his way as El Guindy was identified as the author of this paragraph.[31] However, the British delegate insisted that he was 'unable to accept the conclusions contained in paragraph 6' and attached a reservation to the report of the Sub-Committee that recognized this fact. The Government of India

[29] Ibid. 127.
[30] 'Draft Report Concerning Indian Hemp', in *Records of the Second Opium Conference*, ii. 318.
[31] *Records of the Second Opium Conference*, vol. i, 7 Feb. 1925, p. 222.

representative went even further than this, offering a long and detailed objection to the paragraph. He concluded that the Government of India would honour international agreements designed to restrict and control the smuggling of cannabis into countries where the use of the drugs was forbidden. However, it would not accept 'the suggestions put forward by Sub-Committee F in so far as they affect the methods of internal restriction applied by the various Governments in India'.[32]

This latter point was the key to understanding the British and the India Office rejection. The proposal contained in paragraph 6 on cannabis of Sub-Committee F was not worded so as simply to restrict international movements of the drug in order to prevent smuggling between nations. It was in fact drafted in such a way as to be generally applicable, both in matters of international regulation and of domestic policy. Here then was the application of the controversial American principle that they were pursuing on the issue of opium, that the League of Nations could bind sovereign governments to treaties that imposed on them obligations to change internal laws and to enact internal policies. As already mentioned, this was controversial as it implied that the government of a given nation would no longer be the only authority in that territory, as it would no longer be the only source of legislation and policy, because the League of Nations would be devising programmes that governments would be obliged to enact for their domestic population whether they liked it or not. The Egyptian proposal that was the recommendation of Sub-Committee F on cannabis tacitly recognized and accepted the principle of the American approach to drugs even where the rest of the Conference had yet to decide on its legitimacy. The Government of India had spotted this and had made its point that it would not accept the suggestion that the League of Nations might dictate to a government the policies that it should or should not adopt in relation to its subjects.

When Sub-Committee F reported back to the main Conference on hashish the chairman was at pains to stress that the recommendation was simply 'technical' and in no way was meant to 'suggest any means of introducing an international prohibition'[33] but the Government of India and the British had elected to take no chances by including their objections

---

[32] 'Indian Hemp: Note by the Indian Delegation', in *Records of the Second Opium Conference*, ii. 319.
[33] *Records of the Second Opium Conference*, vol. i, 12 Feb. 1925, p. 262.

in the text of the Sub-Committee's report.[34] El Guindy was in effect trying to take the Conference as far as the Americans wanted it to go on opium but on the issue of cannabis. Indeed, the refusal of many of the rest of the delegations to countenance such an agreement and extension of the League's powers resulted in the Americans walking out of the Conference on 6 February 1925. It was El Guindy and the Egyptian delegation however that continued to fight the American corner in their absence. During the key debate on the issue on 10 February it was El Guindy alone that stood to argue for the American proposal in its pure state.[35]

If the Egyptian delegate had been sincere in pursuing these agendas then he was to be disappointed. The American proposal, in their absence and despite his lonely defence, was qualified and compromised out of all recognition and certainly was not passed in the form they had advocated. Similarly the recommendations on cannabis of Sub-Committee F that El Guindy had authored and from which the British and the Government of India delegates had demurred were obscured and watered down when they came under the scrutiny of those drafting on the subject for inclusion in the Treaty. El Guindy was one of those charged with coming up with a draft section for inclusion in the Treaty and seems to have argued with some tenacity as the chairman of the Sub-Committee convened to look at matters relating to an agreement on Indian hemp took the very unusual step of publicly rapping his colleague for the 'somewhat uncompromising insistence'[36] with which he approached the issue of trade in cannabis and its preparations. When the final draft did appear there were no sweeping references to hemp resin not being 'produced, sold, traded in etc. under any circumstances whatsoever'[37] and there was no sign of the stipulation that 'the use of Indian hemp and the preparations derived therefrom may only be authorised for medical and scientific purposes'. These, of course, were the statements that had so upset the British and the Government of India.

Instead, what there was read as follows.

---

[34] It was the Government of India that took the initiative here and the British delegation followed its lead. A telegram to Sir Malcolm Delevingne from the Secretary of State for the Foreign Office dispatched on the morning of 13 February 1925 instructed him to 'lend your full support to proposal of Indian delegation'. It was felt necessary to have Delevingne instructed in this manner as the Government of India delegates understood that Sir Malcolm was 'personally in favour of the Sub-Committee draft with the possible addition of the words 'so far as the circumstances of each country permit'.

[35] *Records of the Second Opium Conference* vol. i, 10 Feb. 1925, pp. 236–49.

[36] Ibid., 14 Feb. 1925, p. 301.

[37] 'Draft Report Concerning Indian Hemp', ibid. ii. 318.

Chapter IV Article 11

1. In addition to the provisions of Chapter V[38] of the present Convention which shall apply to Indian hemp and the resin prepared from it the Contracting Parties undertake:

a. To prohibit the export of the resin obtained from Indian hemp and the ordinary preparations of which the resin forms the base (such as hashish, esrar, chiras, djamba) to countries which have prohibited their use, and, in cases where export is permitted, to require the production of a special import certificate issued by the Government of the importing country stating that the importation is approved for the purposes specified in the certificate and that the resin or preparations will not be reexported.

b. Before issuing an export authorisation under Article 13 of the present Convention, in respect of Indian hemp, to require the production of a special import certificate issued by the Government of the importing country and stating that the importation is approved and is required exclusively for medical or scientific purposes.

2. The Contracting Parties shall exercise an effective control of such a nature as to prevent the illicit international traffic in Indian hemp and especially in the resin.[39]

In addition to this, Chapter III of the Convention decreed that Contracting Parties would 'enact effective laws or regulations to limit exclusively to medical and scientific purposes the manufacture, import, sale, distribution, export and use of... Galenical preparations (extract and tincture) of Indian hemp'.[40]

However, when El Guindy's original position is considered, and when it is recalled that cannabis was not initially on the agenda and was the subject of a delayed and neglected general inquiry on the part of the Advisory Committee, the progress that he made seems remarkable. He himself admitted at one point that 'my main point was that hashish ought to be included in the list of narcotics', and he had achieved this. He had done this by cleverly playing the politics of the Conference. He had deliberately adopted the position in Sub-Committee F of authoring a recommendation that was as extreme as the American position on opium in advocating that the League of Nations formulate a policy that implied interference in the domestic politics of nation states. This had given him a bargaining position from which to make compromises that would bring him nearer to his true objective of simply including cannabis substances in the laws on international trade in drugs. He had also cultivated the support of

---

[38] This related to international trade and the export/import licensing system.

[39] 'Second Opium Conference Convention Final Act', in *Records of the Second Opium Conference*, ii. 507.

[40] Ibid. 505.

the Americans, both through his espousal of their proposals and also in sharing their determined resistance to British attempts to control the agenda. This ensured that he had powerful allies for his cause. He also lobbied hard and sought support from a range of other delegates. Indeed, by offering up the cannabis issue as a diversion from the central issue of the meeting he found the support of countries such as China and Turkey who were eager for the opportunity to focus attention away from their own positions on opium. The former, due to political division at home, was under criticism for failing to meet its international obligations. The latter, as one of the world's key producers, was keen to avoid incurring any international obligations. El Guindy had manipulated the Geneva meeting so that cannabis found itself on the lists of dangerous substances that were subjected to the international laws of the International Opium Convention.

EXPLAINING EL GUINDY AND THE EGYPTIAN AGENDA

While it is possible to trace the ways in which El Guindy and the Egyptian delegates managed to foist cannabis on to the agenda of the emerging international drugs regulatory system, the League of Nations records do not explain quite why it was that they were so keen to do this. A general concern with cannabis can be traced in Egyptian government for centuries, but El Guindy's sudden assertiveness about the subject and indeed the solutions to the problem that he described so vividly seem to have had rather more contemporary origins. It may well be the case that while the British colonial officials of the Government of India were vigorously opposing his assertions, other branches of Britain's imperial administration were unwittingly supplying him both with his evidence and with his arguments.

Cannabis had been widely used in Egyptian society since medieval times and European observers noted that preparations of the hemp plant were still common in the nineteenth century. Lay medication was popular in Egypt, where it was commented that 'it is worth remarking about the acquaintance the inhabitants of Egypt have with a great quantity of drugs and with their empirically therapeutic usage'.[41] Important among these drugs, noted another French physician, was hashish, which was used as a tonic to stimulate good health rather than to fight illness and which was consumed much as Europeans used fermented liquors.[42] In other words, as

[41] Charles Cuny writing in 1853, quoted in L. Kuhnke, *Lives at Risk: Public Health in Nineteenth Century Egypt* (University of California Press, Berkeley, 1990), 28.
[42] Pierre-Charles Rouyer quoted ibid. 29.

was the case in India, cannabis was seen as both a useful medicine and a pleasant intoxicant.

For as long as cannabis drugs had been used in North Africa they had been frowned upon by the more puritanical or authoritarian of the local elites. Misgivings over intoxicants had been a feature of Islamic law and of Islamic states since the medieval period and at one point users of cannabis in Egypt had faced having their teeth pulled out as punishment for indulgence in the drug.[43] From the nineteenth century onwards the concern of the authorities had been focused in legislation. Napoleon's government in Egypt had tried to forbid the use of cannabis by regulation. The French feared that their soldiers were taking rather too freely to the local intoxicants and that this would impair their effectiveness. After the departure of the French, the Egyptian government passed its own laws in 1868,[44] which were modified at regular intervals after that date. In 1879 it was decided that 'the cultivation, sale, importation or attempt to import haschisch will be punished by a fine of 200 tariff piastres per oke' and all 'boats, carriages, beasts of burden, instruments and any materials whatever which may have served for transporting haschisch, as well as any merchandise used to wrap it up in order to conceal it and facilitate its introduction shall be confiscated'.[45]

The commitment of the Egyptian government in the nineteenth century to trying to prohibit cannabis use in the local population may simply have been an updated rendering of medieval attempts to curb consumption. However, a couple of features of Egyptian history in this period may well be important in explaining the revived interest in the issue. The nineteenth century saw the rise of the government of Mohamed Ali Pasha in 1803 and from then onwards various attempts were made to reform the country and to modernize it along western lines. One of the key issues in this process of modernization was health, as 'Mohamed Ali's drive for an effective military force, as well as for economic development, required a minimum man-

[43] A. M. Khalifa, 'Traditional Patterns of Hashish Use in Egypt', in Rubin, *Cannabis and Culture*, 199. The problem with an understanding of exactly what Islamic legislators and jurists were discussing when it comes to narcotics and stimulants is that the words 'Hashish' (cannabis sativa), 'banj' (drugs), and 'afyūn' (opium) are often lumped together without a precise definition of these terms. Hashish is not however mentioned in the Qur'an or indeed in the oldest Islamic legal texts. For details of this see F. Rosenthal, *The Herb: Hashish Versus Medieval Muslim Society* (Brill, Leiden, 1971).

[44] 'The Policy of Indian Hemp Drug Administration', in *Report of the Indian Hemp Drugs Commission* (Simla, 1894), i. 270.

[45] 'Government of Egypt Decree of March 10 1884' in Reports from Her Majesty's Representatives in Egypt, Greece and Turkey on Regulations affecting the Importation and Sale of Haschisch, in *Parliamentary Papers*, 89 (1893–4), 301.

power level that he soon saw threatened by serious chronic and endemic diseases'.[46] Cannabis use, which was widespread in local society, may well have been drawn into these debates about how to produce a healthy army and workforce, as indeed it was elsewhere.[47] In fact one of Ali's strategies for dealing with the health issue in the country was to found in 1827 a medical school on western lines that was so successful that within half a century 'a medical profession had clearly come into existence in Egypt, one whose members practiced modern Western medicine based on long years of studying and training'.[48] The rise of a modern medical profession in other countries was one of the key elements in increasingly hostile attitudes on the part of the authorities to unregulated consumption of drugs. In England, for example, it was the doctors that campaigned against opium substances in the nineteenth century. Preparations that were freely available for self-medication were seen as rivals to medical expertise, as individuals would not bother consulting a doctor if they felt that they could simply purchase a tried and trusted remedy over the counter. As doctors formed professional bodies these campaigned for control over such pills and potions using the argument that as well-trained practitioners they knew better than the lay person about what ought and ought not to be taken as medicine. It was for this reason that the General Medical Council and the Pharmaceutical Society saw to it that opium preparations were brought under increasing control in Victorian England.[49]

If Islamic misgivings about intoxicants, Egypt's modernizing government, and the rise of a westernised medical profession there provide the context of the country's laws on cannabis in the nineteenth century, they do not explain the particulars of El Guindy's spectacular performance in Geneva. After all, there had been plenty of evidence gathered that Egypt's attempts to control consumption of cannabis preparations among its population was a failure long before he presented the subject in 1924. For example, Lord Cromer wrote from Cairo in 1892 that 'the main facts of the case are very simple. On the one hand the importation and use of haschisch is forbidden by law. On the other hand, it is notorious that the

[46] L. Kuhnke, *Lives at Risk*, 12.

[47] See the discussion of South Africa in n. 18 above. For more on Mohamed Ali Pasha's policies of industrialization and militarization see K. Fahmy, 'The Era of Muhammad Ali Pasha', in M. Daly (ed.), *The Cambridge History of Egypt*, vol. ii (Cambridge University Press, Cambridge, 1998), 161–3.

[48] A. El Azhary Sonbol, *The Creation of a Medical Profession in Egypt, 1800–1922* (Syracuse University Press, New York, 1991), 134

[49] See V. Berridge, *Opium and the People: Opiate Use and Drug Control Policy in Nineteenth and Early Twentieth Century England* (Free Association Books, London, 1999), 113–22.

drug is largely imported and very generally used. It would, under any circumstances, be very difficult to stop haschisch being smuggled into the country.'[50] At no point however had the Egyptian authorities tried to force it upon the agenda of the international drugs meetings as it began to emerge after 1909.

El Guindy's performance in 1924 can in fact be seen as a direct consequence of British imperial interest in the issue of international cannabis smuggling in the 1920s. After the First World War the Government of India, the Governor of the Seychelles, and the British Consul in what was then Abyssinia became caught up in one of the longest-running drug smuggling cases of the immediate post-war period. H. G. de Monfreid, a Frenchman described as an 'adventurer [who] is reputed, probably with truth, to be engaged in gun running and other illicit forms of enterprise', was tracked by the British imperial authorities after he purchased 240 bags of cannabis in Bombay. He later cheerfully admitted that his intention was to smuggle this into Egypt, and indeed confessed that he had been dealing in illicit cannabis substances destined for the country since 1915.[51]

Interest in this case was such that the Colonial Office compiled dossiers on it and regularly supplied information to the British administrators in Egypt itself.[52] Because of this stream of information from across the empire about cannabis smugglers it may well have been they who alerted the local authorities there to the activities of de Monfreid, as the Egyptian police reported in March 1924 that acting 'on information supplied to them' they had succeeded in thwarting some but not all of the smuggling activities. Aware that Egypt was caught up in this large-scale illicit trade the British in Cairo decided to make their own assessment of the situation there. In February 1924 the European Department of the Ministry of the Interior stated that 'the desirability of international cooperation for the control of hashish led to investigations being made in Egypt on the whole question of hashish traffic'. A report was compiled that Lord Allenby forwarded to London in April 1924.

The document was a lengthy investigation of the extent of cannabis use in Egypt. It suggested the complete failure of existing regulations to have an impact on hashish consumption in the country. The key problem identified was the ease of supply. The routes by which the drug came to be in the

[50] Reports from Her Majesty's Representatives in Egypt, Greece and Turkey on Regulations Affecting the Importation and Sale of Haschisch, in *Parliamentary Papers* 89 (1893–4), 294.

[51] H. de Monfreid, *Pearls, Arms and Hashish* (Gollancz, London, 1930), 284–349.

[52] The correspondence between London and Egypt on the case can be found in PRO CO 323/973/9 and other details are available in PRO CO 530/111.

country were varied and difficult to detect. The report noted for example that 'when sent on steamers from Greece and Syria it is put in rubber bags and dropped overboard near the coast: the bags are marked by a float and are picked up by agents afterwards', and it had also found that 'along the coast west of Alexandria or East of Port Said it is landed in small boats and carried inland by Bedouin on camels'. There was a hint of despair as the report noted the many ways in which the drug found its way into the country: 'hashish has been found in the middle of cotton goods from Manchester, it is put in bundles of newspapers from abroad, it is hidden inside imported goods of all kinds such as tins of petroleum, bricks, mill-stones, marble columns, hollow bedsteads, barrels of olives, looking glasses etc.' and even 'sometimes it is made up to resemble the inner soles of boots and the smugglers merely walk ashore with it'. The drug originated in India, Turkey, Greece, and Syria and once in Egypt it was consumed in a variety of ways. The ordinary folk smoked it mixed with molasses and tobacco in a 'goza' or pipe made of coconut-shell. The better off smoked it in cigarettes or ate it as a sweet mixed with spices and honey or sugar. Occasionally it was taken in coffee.

A number of agencies were responsible for policing the trade in the drugs, including the Coast Guard, the Customs officials, and the City Police. The failure of these groups to prevent the trade was blamed on the size of Egypt's borders, on the ease with which the drugs were concealed, and on corruption: 'that collusion exists between the smugglers and some of the employees of the above administrations can hardly be denied; nor is it surprising in view of the enormous profits accruing from the sale of hash-ish'. Indeed, even where smugglers were caught the penalties seemed insuffi-cient, and the report felt that there were special problems in cases where the criminals were foreigners. Under colonial regulations, the western suspect was subject not to Egyptian courts but to the jurisdiction of his country's consular court. The report diplomatically noted that in these circumstances 'it is believed that a condemnation is difficult to obtain'.

The conclusion of the report made it clear that 'it is practically impos-sible to keep hashish out of Egypt'. It was adamant that the only way to improve the situation was to focus on stopping the supply from getting to the country in the first place. The onus was put on international cooper-ation to achieve this. In the first place, the report advocated approaching the Capitulary Powers in order to have their nationals subjected to the same laws as Egyptians. Secondly it noted that 'the import of hashish into Egypt might be reduced if the question was taken up by the League of Nations and hashish was included in the International Opium Convention [as] it is extremely difficult for one country like Egypt to fight single-handed against a noxious drug the traffic of which is openly tolerated in other countries'.[53] The report ended on the conclusion that 'it is suggested therefore that the League of Nations should consider hashish traffic as an international affair and should try to persuade its members to make dealing in or consuming the drug a crime punishable by severe penalties'.

It is worth bearing in mind the fact that these recommendations almost exactly anticipated El Guindy's agenda, and even his language, at the Second Conference, which itself came just over six months after the report. It is also important to consider the fact that the report was made available to Egyptian administrators as it was forwarded to the Director-General of Public Security in Cairo. In this light it seems likely that this is the source of the Egyptian assault on the Geneva Conference in 1924. Indeed, one of the reasons why El Guindy and his delegation would have seized on the document with such enthusiasm is provided in a cautionary note found on the Foreign Office copy of the report in London. Malcolm Delevingne, the British member of the Advisory Committee, saw this dispatch from Lord Allenby and noted that it was 'a very interesting report'. However, he scribbled the argument on the cover of the dossier that it was 'one that for the present we can keep to ourselves'. His reason for this was that he had no intention of providing 'a stick to beat the Capitulary Powers' to those opposed to European interference in Egyptian affairs. The British had after all governed Egypt directly between 1882 and 1922 and retained an informal presence in the country's affairs until after the Second World War, and were perfectly aware of the fact that the country was being swamped with smuggled cannabis and that its laws on the subject throughout this period had failed, and yet they had not bothered to do much about it. In a political climate where Britain's colonial record on drugs was the subject of such scrutiny, another failure would damage both the moral authority of the imperial presence in Egypt[54] and the bargaining position of the British in the international drugs debates. El Guindy's focus on the cannabis issue at the Second Opium Conference may well have stemmed from a genuine concern about the drug. However, many of his facts and most of his agenda seem to have come from a British report and his enthusiasm for

[53] PRO HO 144/6073 Hashish: Traffic and Consumption in Egypt 2 Apr. 1924.

[54] Although the Protectorate had formally ended in 1922 the British still reserved four areas of Egypt's government to its own officers: British imperial communications, defence, foreign interests in Egypt, and the Sudan. As such it maintained a presence in Egyptian administration and politics until 1956. See M. Daly, 'The British Occupation 1882–1922' in Daly (ed.), *Cambridge History of Egypt*, ii. 251.

the subject would have been bolstered by the knowledge that the issue was one that would damage his country's former colonial masters. He had, after all, made a point of announcing his presence at the Opium Conference with the acidic reminder that 'this is the first time that Egypt has been represented by a purely Egyptian delegation at an international conference'.[55]

The argument that the position taken by El Guindy at Geneva was actually founded on British sources is made even more compelling when the scientific basis of the Egyptian argument is considered. El Guindy's dramatic announcements on the mental health implications of cannabis use in Egypt had had a considerable impact on the assembled delegates as he was able to support these with statistics: 'illicit use of hashish is the principal cause of most of the cases of insanity occurring in Egypt ... generally speaking, the proportion of cases of insanity caused by the use of hashish varies from 30 to 60 percent of the total number occurring in Egypt'. Similar evidence made up part of the official 'Memorandum with Reference to Haschiche as it Concerns Egypt' that was submitted by the delegation in support of El Guindy's speeches. However, this time the figure was even more alarming: 'about 70% of insane people in lunatic asylums in Egypt are haschiche eaters or smokers'.[56]

In all of the Egyptian campaigning this was the only material that was produced that might be considered 'medical' or 'scientific' evidence. It is interesting to note then that the Egyptian Lunacy Department, from which these statistics would have been drawn, had been the personal fiefdom of an Englishman for over a quarter of a century between 1895 and 1923. John Warnock was appointed by the Public Health Department in Cairo in 1895 at a time when Egypt was an established part of the British Empire. He had been working in the British asylum system for almost a decade by this time and was seen as the ideal man to reform the Abbasiya Asylum. He remained at the task for twenty-eight years. During this time he expanded the existing institution, built a new hospital, drafted laws on mental illness in Egypt, and created a whole new department dedicated to lunacy within the colonial Ministry of the Interior. By the time he retired almost 2,500 Egyptians were being treated at any one time within the units of the Lunacy Department.

He seems to have developed little attachment to the place that was to be his home for such a large part of his life. He admitted that he did not study written Arabic and that he found it 'impossible to learn all the tongues

---

[55] *Records of the Second Opium Conference*, vol. i, 20 Nov. 1924, pp. 39–40.
[56] PRO HO 144/6073 Egyptian Proposal for Inclusion of Hashish 12 Dec. 1924.

necessary to converse with all the patients and their friends' and his grasp of the vernacular was such that he could only 'make my wants known and give orders'. The country exhausted him and by 1916 he had to take a long leave from the stress of work in Egypt that had been exacerbated by the presence of shell-shocked soldiers from the African campaigns of the First World War. He contemptuously dismissed Egyptian political ambitions after the war and noted that 'self-determination was proving to be an infectious mental disorder'.[57] Yet despite this apparent lack of sympathy with the society around him he felt sure that he could locate the chief cause of insanity in the Egyptian population. This was the use of cannabis.

His first year at the asylum was a particularly trying period. He arrived in February 1895 and noted the following difficulties.

Besides the almost complete lack of funds, my total ignorance of Arabic, and the total ignorance of patients and staff of any language but Arabic, prevented my doing anything for some time. I was unable even to tell the servant to shut the door or to ask a patient his name. I had no interpreter. However, after some time I found a patient who could write English and for a while he was employed in translating Arabic letters etc. until it was discovered that he interpolated numerous mis-statements founded on his delusions. In those days an English or French-speaking clerk was not available. For a time I could only look on and guess at what was going on in most matters.

Yet despite the range of difficulties in gathering accurate details about patients that included problems of translation, problems of deliberate misinformation, problems of communicating with staff, and a reliance on guess work, Warnock claimed that he was able to produce an authoritative account of the causes of mental illness in the asylum within ten months of his arrival. This was reported as 'The Cairo Asylum: Dr Warnock on Hasheesh Insanity by TS Clouston MD Edinburgh', which was published in the *Journal of Mental Science* in 1896. This was a summary of Warnock's observations of the asylum statistics that his hospital had generated in the period from his arrival at the hospital in February to the end of 1895. These statistics were central to the argument and after noting such numbers as 'in 41 percent of all his male patients hasheesh alone or combined with alcohol caused the disease', he concluded that 'I have no doubt that in quite a number of cases there hasheesh is the chief if not the only cause of the mental disease'. He went on to note the clinical features of this 'Hasheesh Insanity' that included 'an elated, reckless state, in which optical hallucin-

----

[57] J. Warnock, 'Twenty-Eight Years' Lunacy Experience in Egypt (1895–1923)', *Journal of Mental Science*, 70 (1924), 233–61.

ations and delusions that devils possess the subject frequently exist' or even 'terrifying hallucinations, fear of neighbours, outrageous conduct, continual restlessness and talking, sleeplessness, exhaustion, marked incoherence and complete absorption in insane ideas'. The statistics, and the exotic location, seem to have been enough to convince T. S. Clouston, who exclaimed, 'such are the latest words in regard to hasheesh and its insanity'.[58] Clouston, as was noted in Chapter 4, had developed an interest in cannabis back in the 1860s through his experiments with hemp drugs as a cure for mental illness.

Despite Warnock's frank admissions that he had very little idea of what was going on upon his arrival in Egypt and indeed had no reliable means of remedying this situation beyond hazarding a few guesses of his own and trying to interpret the lunatic translations of his delusional clerk, it seems that he was happy to jump to conclusions about the cause of illness among a large proportion of his patients within twelve months of his taking up the post. He may well have read an earlier report on Egyptian mental illness— he had certainly seen this by the end of his career as he noted it in his 1924 article, which argued that 'with the men the attack of insanity was attributed in nearly all cases to one of three causes, the use of hashish, some disappointment or grief, and religious excitement. Of these, the first is by far the most frequent.'[59] Whatever was the case, these were conclusions that he stuck to. In 1903 he published a lengthy account of his observations at the asylum. Again he relied on numerical evidence to make his point: 'in Egypt, statistics are available since the year 1895. During the six years 1896–1901 out of 2564 male cases of insanity admitted to the Egyptian Asylum at Cairo, 689 were attributed to the abuse of hasheesh, i.e. nearly 27 per cent.' He quoted statistics from India to make the comparison: 'between 1882 and 1892 Indian hemp caused 25 to 35 per cent of the insanity in Bengal asylums'—even though the reliability of these numbers had been challenged by the Indian Hemp Drugs Commission itself. He was at pains to refute the conclusions of the IHDC and emphasized that 'my experience does not confirm the Indian Commission's belief that cannabis indica only sometimes causes insanity. In Egypt it frequently causes insanity.' He was keen to stress that his statistics—and remember that they were his statistics, as he admits that the collection of this data only began in 1895 when he arrived—were entirely dependable. He did this by claiming

---

[58] T. Clouston, 'The Cairo Asylum: Dr Warnock on Hasheesh Insanity', *Journal of Mental Science*, 42 (1896), 793–4.

[59] A. Urquhart and S. Tuke, 'Two Visits to the Cairo Asylum, 1877 and 1878', *Journal of Mental Science*, 25 (1879–80), 43–53.

that each patient counted as a sufferer of hashish insanity was correctly diagnosed. He did not believe police reports of hashish use nor did he give much credence to relatives of the patient. Indeed, he did not believe the patients themselves, noting that 'excited protests and denials of the habit are known by experience to indicate a hardened hasheesh smoker'. Instead he relied on his own intuition and repeated questioning of the patients until a confession was obtained.

Quite how reliable this method was of establishing that a case was one of cannabis use is worth considering. In 1895 he stated that he thought that one of the key symptoms of weak-mindedness caused by hashish insanity was that 'they deny the use of hasheesh'. He made it clear in 1903 that 'as the mental state of the patient improves he is again questioned about hasheesh and before discharge he is invited to give full details of his habit'. It seems then that procedures in Warnock's hospital encouraged inmates to confess to use of cannabis preparations, as the final hurdle before release was another interrogation on the subject of cannabis use by a doctor who admitted that he could consider a denial of the habit as a symptom of problems of mental illness.

In fact his conclusions themselves are more wide ranging than they have a right to be. Based on his experience of cases at the asylum that he believed to be caused by cannabis use he made sweeping observations such as 'the use of cannabis indica in Egypt seems to have graver mental and social results than in India and is responsible for a large amount of insanity and crime in this country'. However, he also admitted that 'as to whether excessive use of hemp drugs is commoner here than in India I can give no opinion, but many thousands use it daily here', and indeed went further in noting that while 'many thousands smoke hasheesh only a comparatively few suffer from grave toxic symptoms'.[60] In other words he made broad generalizations about cannabis use and cannabis users that were meant to apply to all users in all of Egypt despite the fact that he saw only a small proportion of them at the hospitals. The issue of whether this was a representative proportion of the cannabis users in the country never seems to have troubled him and he broadened his conclusions drawn from the troubled individuals at the asylum to apply to thousands of ordinary Egyptians that took hashish and yet never became subjects of his scrutiny. In short, his method of establishing that an individual at his hospital was a cannabis user was suspect and the conclusions that he drew about cannabis use in general were based simply on the small sample of all of Egypt's many users

---

[60] J. Warnock, 'Insanity from Hasheesh', *Journal of Mental Science*, 49 (1903), 96–110.

that had ended up in his hospital. Much as in India in the nineteenth century, the habits indulged in by much of the local population were condemned by colonial doctors who had no idea what was going on outside of the walls of the hospital and to whom it never occurred that a small band of lunatics could in no way be considered a representative sample on which to base observations about wider society.

Whatever the veracity of Warnock's thesis it remains the case that it was this British medical officer that was churning out statistics and judgements on cannabis use in Egypt for over a quarter of a century before Dr El Guindy used just such statistics and judgements to throw cannabis on to the agenda of the international drugs regulatory system. It seems a rich irony of imperialism that the determination of the British and the British Indian delegations to resist the intrusion of cannabis into the regulatory system in 1925 was undermined by an Egyptian position that is likely to have been established because of a report authored by British officials in the country in 1924 on the issue and which was bolstered by the statistics of a British medical officer who had been building Cairo's lunatic asylum for over twenty-five years. The many tentacles of the empire seem to have become entangled on the issue of cannabis.

8

'An outcome of cases that have come before the police courts of the use of hashish': DORA, the First World War, and the Domestic Drug Scares of the 1920s

DRUGS AND BRITAIN IN THE 1920S

On 11 May 1916 the Army Council passed an order that forbade the sale of Indian hemp to any member of the Armed Forces unless the transaction was ordered by a doctor or pharmacist on a written prescription that was dated and signed by him and marked 'not to be repeated'. This order was also applied to cocaine and opium, codeine, heroin, and morphine. However, later in the year when similar restrictions were extended to the rest of the population in the Defence of the Realm Act (DORA) it seems that Indian hemp was not on the list of substances to be controlled. Indeed, with the end of hostilities the 1916 DORA wartime regulations were placed on a permanent footing in the Dangerous Drugs Acts of 1920 and 1923 but once again cannabis was not caught up in the regulations and it remained freely available and unaffected by these new controls.

However, in 1924 Indian hemp was proposed by the Pharmaceutical Society for addition to the list of substances that were to be regulated by another set of drugs regulations. The Poisons Acts had existed since the nineteenth century as a means of controlling the population's access to a range of toxic substances and once the Privy Council accepted the Pharmaceutical Society's suggestion cannabis was officially classified as a poison. This was the first time that there had been legal restrictions on the sale and possession of cannabis preparations to the general public in the United Kingdom. Under these restrictions only a chemist could sell substances that contained cannabis and then they could only be sold to an individual known to the chemist or to someone that was accompanied by an individual known to the chemist. The details of the purchaser and the transaction were noted in the poisons register kept at the shop. The container for the purchase had to carry a label with the name of the drug and the proportion of the drug to other ingredients and had to have the word 'POISON' spelt out, the latter in red letters or set against a red background. These new restrictions on the sale of cannabis came into effect in 1925.

It was in that year that the League of Nations Opium Convention discussed in the previous chapter was ratified in Parliament. This meant that cannabis could not be imported or exported without a licence and could only be exported to a country in which the government permitted imports. It also meant that certain preparations of cannabis, the pharmaceutically manufactured extract and tincture of Indian hemp medicines, were available only for medical and scientific usage. It also gave the government the power to pass further regulations on cannabis and coca leaves if it saw fit to do so. This it duly did in 1928 with the Coca Leaves and Indian Hemp Regulations. These stipulated that the right to sell or possess preparations of cannabis was reserved for pharmacists, doctors, dentists, and vets and those who had been granted a licence to possess the drugs, such as wholesale drugs merchants supplying the pharmaceutical trade. The ordinary citizen could only possess cannabis or preparations of cannabis if he or she had been prescribed it by one of the above.

The 1920s then was the decade in which cannabis first found itself the subject of official restrictions and regulations in Britain. The origins of the international controls that were incorporated into UK law in 1925 were explored in the previous chapter in the politics of opium and in Britain's imperial relationships. However, even this brief survey suggests that there is also a domestic history of government interest in cannabis, and the Army Council and the Pharmaceutical Society have been mentioned as examples of groups that turned their attention to Indian hemp in this period. This chapter will explain why cannabis suddenly found itself the subject of concern and a focus for the authorities during and after the First World War in Britain.

THE FIRST WORLD WAR AND DRUGS

By the end of the First World War the military authorities had seen to it that it was far from easy for a soldier to get himself intoxicated and, indeed, the civil authorities, taking their cue from the generals, had done their best to extend these restrictions to the rest of the population. Alcohol was the first target: 'we are fighting Germany, Austria and Drink; and as far as I can see the greatest of these three deadly foes is Drink,' declared Lloyd George in 1915.[1] As early as August 1914 the military assumed the right to close public-houses and to restrict opening hours in garrison towns. These powers were quickly adopted by the civil authorities and in 1915 the Central Control Board (Liquor Traffic) was established. This reduced public-house opening times from up to seventeen hours a day to five and a half hours on weekdays with a compulsory afternoon ban on selling alcohol and an evening closing time of 9.30 p.m. The government also placed restrictions on the output of brewing companies and in 1916 legislation limited the amount of beer produced to 85 per cent of the previous year's 30 million barrels. This was further reduced in 1917 to 28 per cent of pre-war levels and in that year only 14 million barrels were produced. The government also insisted that the brewers make beers with lower alcohol content, drinks that came to be known as 'Government Ale'. Indeed, in some key centres of munitions manufacture such as Carlisle, the government nationalized the breweries in order to impose tight control on production.[2]

Drugs were to be the next target. Stories began to circulate in the press about the use of opium and cocaine amongst off-duty soldiers in London and a murky connection between these troops, prostitutes, and foreign drugs dealers hinted at exotic pleasures and alien vices at a time when troops were expected to be focused on the rigours of fighting. Such were the fears that the Allied armies were being undermined by foreign suppliers of drugs that the authorities acted on 11 May 1916 and passed an Order in the name of the Army Council that prohibited the sale of a range of drugs to any member of the Armed Forces unless the transaction was sanctioned by a doctor or pharmacist on a written prescription that had been dated and signed by him and marked 'not to be repeated'. The Order was targeted at the main temptations of opium and cocaine but included a list of other

[1] Quoted in T. Gourvish and R. Wilson, *The British Brewing Industry, 1830–1980* (Cambridge University Press, Cambridge, 1994), 318.
[2] Ibid. 317–27.

substances including codeine, heroin, and morphine. Tucked away on the list was cannabis.

Quite why hemp should have merited a mention on this list is difficult to ascertain as the records do not reveal how this list of drugs was drawn up.[3] One possibility would be that the measure was aimed at Indian troops that were in Europe as they had been fighting in France in 1914 and 1915 and particularly at their wounded who had been sent to convalesce in Brighton. It may have been the case that these had formed a market for Indian hemp drugs as Asian sailors visiting the UK were to do in the 1920s.[4] Another explanation would be that the medical authorities of the Indian Army had been consulted and had advised that the drug be added to the list. Whatever was the case restrictions on the supply of cannabis were for the first time imposed on British citizens, in this case on the country's soldiers.

When the civil translation of the restrictions is considered it is even more difficult to explain why Indian hemp deserved a mention in the Army's order. Just as the government had followed the military in adopting restrictions on alcohol, so it chose to adopt the Army's approach on drugs under the Defence of the Realm Act. Regulation 40B was put into place on 28 July 1916, the same day that the government gave itself a raft of emergency powers that included the right to suspend bank holidays and the ability to prosecute anyone melting down gold coins. The aim of the Regulation was twofold, to prevent the supply of drugs to soldiers via civilian intermediaries and to stop opium being smuggled from Britain for sale in China at a time when there was a concern that 'the supplies of opium in the United Kingdom should be adequate for military needs' as painkillers for the wounded. The need to protect UK supplies of opiates seemed urgent given the wartime demand and the evidence that large amounts of the drugs were being smuggled abroad by Chinese traders based in the UK. Documents considered by the government officials charged with formulating Regulation 40B included a dossier of letters translated from the Chinese of a gang of opium smugglers operating between China, Hong Kong, America, and Liverpool. The Chief Constable of Liverpool had written a report detailing his powerlessness under existing laws to stop the preparation of

---

[3] For example the 'Minutes of the Proceedings of and Precis Prepared for the Army Council for the Years 1915 and 1916' (PRO WO 33/881) contains no mention of the drugs issue.

[4] The Home Office was aware that visiting Indian and Arab sailors bought and sold cannabis for their own use in British ports. See PRO HO 144/6073 Hashish: Inclusion in List of Dangerous Drugs 20 Feb. 1924. For more on the experience of Indian troops in Britain in the First World War see D. Omissi, *Indian Voices of the Great War* (Macmillan, Basingstoke, 1999).

opium for smuggling despite the fact that he could identify the houses—32, 42, and 59 Pitt Street and 43 Mersey Street—where the drugs were being prepared by Chinese merchants for export. One opium smuggler, Ko Low, was reputed to have made a profit of £30,000 in 1915 alone and Holt & Company, one of Liverpool's leading shipping companies, insisted in 1916 that 'the illicit traffic in opium has now attained to most formidable dimensions'.[5]

The most detailed restrictions of Regulation 40B were therefore on raw and powdered opium, making it an offence for anyone except medical men, pharmacists, and vets to be in possession of the drugs, to sell them, or indeed to give them away. Cocaine was also included in the list of restricted drugs to prevent prostitutes from supplying it to soldiers. All transactions involving the substances had to be covered by prescriptions. However, Indian hemp was not on the list of drugs covered by Regulation 40B so none of its restrictions applied to cannabis. Indeed, while the military seems to have had a concern with cannabis there is no mention of Indian hemp in the documents left by the government's interdepartmental conference held on the 19 June that was to give rise to Regulation 40B. Although mention was briefly made of 'other pernicious drugs' in the documents, it seems that these were not named and were certainly not considered at any great length. DORA ignored cannabis because cocaine and opium were the targets.

Indeed, when the DORA Regulations and the 1912 Hague Opium Convention recommendations were all put onto a permanent legislative footing in the UK after the War cannabis similarly failed to get a mention in the deliberations of the administrators, medical men, and pharmacists that gathered to formulate policy. The 1920 Dangerous Drugs Act targeted morphine, cocaine, ecgonine, heroin, and medicinal opium and deemed that supply of these drugs and indeed possession of these drugs was illegal unless covered by a medical prescription. The proceedings of the committee that devised these regulations show that the main topics of debate concerned the time consuming nature of the administration involved and the problems associated with forged prescriptions. When drugs were considered by the committee the problems fell into two categories, that of common remedies that would suddenly find themselves outlawed and that of veterinary drugs that contained opium. Certain morphia preparations were allowed to be exempted from the regulations as they were widely used and not believed to be dangerous but all substances containing more than 0.1 per cent cocaine were listed. As for drugs used by vets and other 'cow-doctors' the commit-

[5] PRO PC 8/803 Minute of Inter-Departmental Conference on Opium Traffic.

tee observed that most opiates used on animals were too weak to be affected by the regulations and that anyway 'it was hoped that most of the difficulty in these cases might be got over by the addition to the drug of some denaturant which, while not affecting the medicinal qualities of the preparations, would make them too nauseous for human use'.[6] While this issue of individuals with a craving for farmyard opiates came to occupy the committee passing regulations under the 1920 Dangerous Drugs Act there was no room for consideration of Indian hemp. Cannabis and cannabis preparations were not even discussed by those devising Britain's new post-war drugs laws.

THE POLICE, THE PRESS, PARLIAMENT, AND THE NEW DOPE PERIL

Indeed, cannabis during the war years and in the early 1920s only really registered with the government when it was implicated in British dealings abroad. For example, the Foreign Office had followed the case of Alex Tanti, who was convicted in Cairo in 1914 of living from the proceeds of prostitution and permitting a house of his to be used for the smoking of hashish. On two previous occasions when the Egyptian Courts had tried to close down the café that Tanti owned and where he supplied hashish to customers he had used his nationality to thwart the authorities, declaring on one occasion that 'the place is mine and I am a British subject and I oppose the execution [of the order to close the café]'. When finally the Egyptian authorities reported him to the British he was tried by the Consular Court and sentenced to a year's hard labour for the first offence and three months with hard labour for the drugs crime. He was sent to serve his sentence at the prison on the island of Malta.[7]

After the First World War, a number of British colonial administrations were embroiled in one of the most remarkable drug smuggling cases of the 1920s. H. G. de Monfreid, a Frenchman, had bought 10 tons of cannabis, probably charas, in Bombay in 1922. It was licensed for export to Abyssinia as 'an insecticide' and transported in 240 bags. The first stop on the way to Abyssinia was at the Seychelles, where the suspicion of the British Governor was aroused. Aware that the consignment had potential

---

[6] PRO HO 45/24739 Signed Report of the Committee on the draft regulations under the Dangerous Drugs Act 1920.

[7] PRO FO 841/146 Alexander Tanti for permitting the use and smoking of hashish 25 Apr. 1914

as a source of drugs he forbade its onward journey while he investigated the subject. Having taken almost four months to satisfy himself that he had no grounds to restrict its passage he let it go on its journey, the packages passing through French Somaliland before arriving in Abyssinia. By the time they arrived in Harar 120 of the bags were found to contain organic fertilizer rather than cannabis. The remaining 120 bags were impounded by the authorities in Abyssinia and eventually sent back to French Somaliland for collection by de Monfreid. Once he collected it there it was shipped via Aden to Hamburg and once in Germany it was opened and the remaining 120 bags of cannabis were also found to have suddenly become organic fertilizer—'a plant soil chemically treated on a vegetable fertilising base'. Mystery surrounded the question of where the hemp had gone and how the authorities had managed to lose track of 10 tons of cannabis that they had been monitoring for almost two years between 1922 and 1924. The reason they had been watching the consignment was that de Monfried was a notorious 'adventurer, and is reputed, probably with truth, to be engaged in gun running and other illicit forms of enterprise'. In fact in the First World War he was accused of supplying arms and information to the Turks in the Yemen and it was noted that his wife was a German whose father still lived in Stuttgart. He had been arrested and sentenced for gun running in 1914 and 1915 and also in 1918 but on each occasion the French authorities in Somaliland vouched for him and secured his freedom.

De Monfreid argued that he was in fact the victim of deception. He had exported the Indian hemp because it was an insecticide commonly used in Turkestan, but a gang of Greeks was supposed to have stolen some and smuggled it into Egypt on board the ship of a passing princess while de Monfreid's agent, one Captain Ternel, was alleged to have tried to sell the consignment to an Egyptian syndicate after attempting to bribe the Italian and French consuls on the Seychelles for shipping permits. The British, however, had other evidence. In 1925 the Consulate in Abyssinia wrote that the Frenchman had made such significant profits in 1923 from his part in the illicit trade in cannabis that he had been able to buy a controlling interest in the flour mills and electric lighting works in Dire Dawa. Indeed, de Monfreid had begun to encourage local farmers in Abyssinia to grow Indian hemp for him. He collected the locally grown produce and added it to that which he was obtaining from elsewhere. He then had this raw hemp manufactured into charas and subsequently arranged to smuggle it into Egypt. The British Consul writing in 1925 observed that 'de Monfreid's initial essays in this respect two years ago were so successful that it is hard to believe that he would easily abandon such a lucrative adventure'. De Monfreid later confessed that he had been a cannabis smuggler and complained that the British had harassed him as they had seen him as a competitor to their own drugs supply networks.[8]

There was one group rather closer to home, however, that had become increasingly agitated by cannabis in the early 1920s. It seems that the Metropolitan Police had been advocating that Indian hemp be included on the Dangerous Drugs Act lists as early as 1921. A letter in Home Office files in 1923 from the CID at New Scotland Yard claimed that 'the desirability of including hashish in the regulations under the Dangerous Drugs Act was reported to the Home Office some two years ago' and indeed it went on to observe that 'it is regretted that this drug is not included in the Dangerous Drugs Act. It appears that it has practically the same effect as cocaine and morphine has upon its victims.'[9] The Home Office was dismissive of such exaggerated claims and an official noted after reading the letter that 'no sort of evidence is adduced that there is any real prevalence of the hashish habit or that the habit if acquired has any results subversive of public morality'. The police lobbying therefore failed to have the drugs included on the 1923 revision of the legislation.

However, the issue received a public airing because of a piece of police blundering in London in that year. The case of Thomas Garza and Idris Abdullah showed that there was a trade in cannabis being carried on right in the heart of London. Abdullah was registered with the police as a Soudanese subject and had been employed 'in native costume' as a coffee maker in various West End restaurants. Garza was also employed as a coffee maker at the Trocadero Restaurant on Shaftesbury Avenue and was registered as an Abyssinian. Charles Owen, a detective with the CID at New Scotland Yard, reported his account of a meeting with the two men as follows.

Acting on information received at 4.30pm 8th August 1923, with Detective Dixon I went to 12 Old Compton Street and there saw prisoner Garza outside the street door. I said to him 'are you the person who has some opium to dispose of?' He said 'yes come inside'. Dixon and I followed Garza up the stairs to a back room on the top floor. In this room was the prisoner Abdullah. Garza introduced me to him as the person who wished to purchase opium. Garza then locked the

---

[8] The British information on de Monfreid can be found in PRO CO 323/973/9 and PRO CO 530/111. However, Henri de Monfreid's own account of his cannabis smuggling exploits is available in H. de Monfreid, *Pearls, Arms and Hashish* (Gollancz, London, 1930), 284–349 and in *Hashish: A Smuggler's Tale* (Penguin, London, 1946).

[9] PRO HO 144/6073 Dangerous Drugs Act: Inclusion of Hashish, Bhang and Indian Hemp 21 Aug. 1923.

door at the same time saying 'we must be careful'. I said to him 'have you got any opium here?' Garza replied 'my friend here is a little afraid of you, because he doesn't know you. Last month the police came here and he is suspicious now'.

Garza then held a conversation with Abdullah who after some hesitation unlocked a trunk in front of the window and took from the bottom of the trunk a large cake of brown substance closed in a canvas bag on which was stamped in red a sign of a double eagle with the word 'extra' underlined. Abdullah pointed to this stamp and said 'Bon! Good!' I said to him 'is it good?' Garza then replied 'yes, it is pure Persian opium'. I said 'how much do you expect for this?' Garza said 'ten pounds'. I then sent Detective Dixon to telephone to this Office for the assistance of another Officer and during his absence the prisoners and I conversed on general subjects.

On the return of Detective Dixon I said to Garza 'have you any more opium?' and he replied 'no, but when you like I can get plenty from a friend'. I said 'how much?' and he replied 'I will get you plenty of good Persian opium if you have the money'. I then said 'we are Police Officers, I shall arrest you both for offering to supply opium'. Garza said 'it belongs to a friend and I tried to do him a turn'. Abdullah said 'me lose my work'.

They were conveyed to Marlborough Street Police Station and detained. Later with Detectives Dixon and Sorrell I went to the prisoners' address and there found in a trunk under a window in Abdullah's room (the same room in which I first saw prisoners) four large parcels each containing two similar slabs to that already offered and also a quantity of the same material broken up.

The newspapers were quick to seize on this story and the *Daily Mail* and *The Times* reported it two days later while the *News of the World* picked it up two days after that on 12 August. Under the headline 'Man in a Fez' the latter reported that 'alleged traffickers in "dope" named Idris Abdullah and Thomas Garza were arrested by detectives in Soho on suspicion of trafficking in opium. Before the magistrate at Marlborough Street Abdullah, who is 41, wore a fez; Garza aged 32, is an Italian subject. They were described as coffee makers of Old Compton Street.' The case quickly became controversial as the magistrate at the Police Court in Marlborough Street was rather perturbed by the approach of the detectives. He commented that as the men were to be charged with 'offering to supply raw opium without authority' it was by no means clear that the action of the police in inducing that offer did not 'affect the moral aspect of the case'. Indeed, he accused the police of being morally wrong and stated that he believed that the men would not have offered the opium had they not been asked to do so.

Perhaps more controversial still, however, were the results of tests carried out on the substance that the accused had offered the policemen. Detective

Owen had taken a sample to the Government Analyst who had declared that it was in fact 'a drug manufactured from Indian hemp and was known as Hashish'. The police enlisted a second opinion and called in Mr S. W. Lawson who was the Acting Superintendent of Police in Khartoum. He confirmed that it was hashish and that it was an offence against the Sudan Penal Code to deal in it in that country. He seemed to think however that the hashish was from there. New Scotland Yard decided to give the impression that they had been aware all along that the substance was cannabis and Inspector Walter Burmby declared that 'it has been known to Police for some months past that these two men had been dealing in this drug, which is commonly called opium in the Soudan'. If this had been the case, quite why the detectives would have wanted to arrest the accused would have needed explaining as Garza and Abdullah were simply offering to sell cannabis, something that they were perfectly entitled to do as it was subject to no restrictions at that time. However, the men remained charged with attempting to supply opium and the police insisted that the case go to court. When there it became clear that Abdullah had very limited English so it was impossible to demonstrate that he understood that his colleague, Garza, was offering to supply raw opium. As such the charge against him was withdrawn. Garza was sent for trial at the County of London Sessions on 21 August 1923. His defence was that he was simply acting as an interpreter between Abdullah and the prospective customers and that as such he was not transacting on his own behalf. The jury seems to have been satisfied with this and he was found 'not guilty' of the charge.

The police had arrested Garza and Abdullah for offering to supply cannabis, something which at the time the two men were legally entitled to do; they had then prosecuted them for trying to supply opium and had failed to secure a conviction against either man. Despite all this, they would still not let the matter drop. The solicitors representing the police in the prosecution wrote to the Home Office arguing that 'the facts of this case go to show quite clearly that there is in London a traffic in this stuff, and there can be little doubt that both these men, who were Coffee Makers and Servers in West End Restaurants were supplying this noxious article for consumption in Coffee or otherwise to persons whom they knew to be addicted to the habit of taking it'.

Indeed, it is possible to suspect that the police did not simply argue their case through solicitors and with the Home Office. The newspapers seized on the story and accounts such as that of the *Daily Chronicle* suggest that the police were often very helpful in supplying information. The allegation that there was 'a serious growth in the traffic of hashish, a deadly Eastern drug which induces madness in this country' very closely followed the police line as did the conclusion that 'hashish is being used as freely as dope in this country, the practice is probably of very recent growth, and may be due to the obstacles placed in the way of obtaining cocaine by recent police action'. Other newspapers were less concerned to parrot police opinions but were no less excited about the story. *The Times* on 18 August wrote the story up under the headline 'HASHISH NOT OPIUM: New Turn in Drug-Dealing Case' and reported the prosecution solicitor making the statement that hashish 'was used in that form for exactly the same purposes as heroin, cocaine and morphine. It was a narcotic, an excitant, and irritant and when indulged in to excess it induced madness.' The *Daily Mail* similarly reported this statement and went further, naming the Coventry Restaurant on Regent Street as the place of employment of Abdullah and revealing that hashish 'can be put into a pipe and smoked or put into coffee'. Other headlines included 'The New Dope Peril: Hashish to Come under Dangerous Drugs Act' and 'Hashish: Drug Forgotten by Law' and stories speculated that 'a second amendment to the Dangerous Drugs Act will probably be presented to Parliament by the Home Secretary in the next session as a result of the recent discovery of the omission of the words 'hashish, bhang, or Indian hemp'. One official scribbled the word 'liar!' in the margin of a Home Office copy of the *Daily Mail* from 23 August that claimed that 'a Home Office official stated yesterday that it was not possible at present to announce any decision regarding hashish but that one might be arrived at in the course of the next fortnight'.[10] The combination of exotic substances, mysterious foreigners, and the metropolitan setting of the West End evoked the cocaine scare stories of the wartime period and so proved irresistible to the press.

At first sight it appears that the Home Office was little concerned about the case or indeed about the press coverage, one internal memo suggesting that the reports were evidence of the journalists 'having nothing better to do'. However, cannabis had come to the notice of the officials for other reasons and documents collected by the Home Office show the gathering uncertainty about hashish. The first of these related to a case in South Shields in Northumberland. William Scott, the Chief Constable there in August 1922 had forwarded a pipe and two samples of a substance that his officers had recovered at the house of Mr A. Hamed of 5 Tiny Street.

---

[10] PRO HO 144/6073 Hashish: Traffic Amongst Orientals 6 Sept. 1923 and Dangerous Drugs Act: Inclusion of Hashish, Bhang and Indian Hemp 21 Aug. 1923.

A local chemist had declared that it was neither opium nor hashish and the Chief Constable was rather perplexed as to what had been discovered. The Government Laboratory in London confirmed that it was indeed hashish and that the pipe could be used for smoking either opium or hashish but that in fact it had not been used for either. The Home Office was intrigued by this report from the shores of the North-East and asked in its reply to Scott's letter 'if you should observe the smoking of Hashish to be prevalent in your district'. The Chief Constable replied that it was not and it was explained that Hamed was alleged to have been selling opium to Indians and that the hashish had been found alongside the pipe in the man's coalhouse. The matter does not seem to have proceeded from there.[11] Malcolm Delevingne at the Home Office was satisfied that there was no widespread use of the drugs in South Shields among the local population and observed that the town had 'an Arab Colony'. Indeed, he was sure that the British had not taken to cannabis and that no further restrictions were necessary as 'it is probable that the haschish consumption is confined to Arab, Greek and Lascar seamen [and] it is doubtful whether restrictions would diminish the vice amongst them, who could always smuggle in sufficient for their needs'.[12]

Another curious episode in the Welsh borders, however, caused some doubts about Sir Malcolm's conclusions. While the evidence for either suggestion ultimately seems cloudy, there was for a time the possibility that cannabis was either being smoked with tobacco in the provinces by British youths or that UK cigarette companies were sneaking a little hashish into their ingredients. In the *British Medical Journal* of 22 September 1923 a doctor in Shrewsbury reported on the following house call.

I was summoned one evening to see a young woman who was reported to have become suddenly 'paralysed'. On arrival at the house the mother told me that about two hours previously her daughter had introduced into her nose some tobacco dust after which she had become very giddy and had lost the use of her legs. It appeared that a young man spending the evening with them had induced the girl, and also her sister, by way of a rather foolish joke, to sniff up the dusty tobacco at the bottom of his pouch in the manner of snuff. The sister, aged 17, had shortly afterwards vomited violently and no further untoward symptoms developed in her case. The patient however aged 18 I found in a very curious condition.

He went on to describe the behaviour of the older girl who had evidently taken to the powder rather more enthusiastically than had her younger

---

[11] PRO HO 144/6073 Substance Discovered in Coal House in South Shields 9 Aug. 1922.
[12] PRO HO 144/6073 Hashish: Inclusion in List of Dangerous Drugs 20 Feb. 1924.

sibling. He observed that 'she was lying on a couch, frankly intoxicated (no alcohol had been administered) talking incoherently and giggling in a fatuous manner. She could not move her lower limbs, the feet and lower legs being completely anaesthetic and there was general paraesthesia. The pupils were dilated and the pulse was frequent. She was oblivious to her surroundings unless well shaken when she took some notice and would answer questions.' The medic, with the rather suitable name of Doctor Downer, administered an emetic and large doses of black coffee to combat the effects of whatever it was up her nose and he managed successfully to bring the girl back to her senses.

The doctor had the good sense to take possession of the remains of the substance that had so affected the girl and he took it off to a friend of his in Shrewsbury. Dr Herbert Henstock was a local chemist and, after devising a test of his own, he came to the conclusion that the powder inhaled by the girl was smoking tobacco with '0.66 per cent of solid cannabis indica in the sample, equivalent roughly to about 1 drachm of the BP tincture per ounce of tobacco'.[13] It appeared that Drs Downer and Henstock had discovered cannabis smoking in the heart of Shropshire.

The Times noticed the letter from Dr Downer in the *British Medical Journal* and published a short report of it on the 24 September 1923 under the headline 'Hashish in Tobacco: A Disquieting Case'. It concluded that 'ordinary smoking tobacco may sometimes be contaminated with Indian hemp . . . the continued smoking of even minute quantities of "hashish" is likely to prove exceedingly harmful'.[14] Arthur Fisher MP, while reading the papers at his home in Chichester, had noticed this piece and dashed off a letter the same day to the Ministry of Health insisting that they find out the name of the cigarette that had been analysed by Dr Henstock, that officials should warn the public of that brand's poisonous ingredients, and that a prosecution of the company for adulterating their product should be initiated. Evidently the newspaper article had struck a chord with Fisher as he stated in his letter that 'before this case was found out a Doctor told me he was convinced that there was something now in the tobaccos which was poisonous. He smokes a pipe.' He warned that if the Ministry did not act he 'could get the question asked in the House'.

The Ministry did act although the way in which they pursued the case showed that they were not as convinced as was Fisher that cigarette companies were mixing cannabis in with their tobacco. Dr Downer was con-

---

[13] R. Downer, 'Cannabis Indica in Smoking Tobacco', *British Medical Journal*, 2 (1923), 521.
[14] PRO HO 144/6073 Popular Brand of Tobacco Containing Drug 24 Sept. 1923.

tacted to see if it was possible that the young man who owned the cigarette pouch in which the offending dust had settled was likely to have added the hashish to the tobacco himself. Dr Downer replied that 'the young man [is] quite an unsophisticated person whom [*sic*], I feel sure, had never even heard of cannabis indica'. The Ministry then contacted the Customs and Excise to see if they had any information about the adulteration of cigarettes with cannabis. The latter decided to test a number of brands of cigarettes to check the story. The Government Laboratory failed to find cannabis in any of the samples and indeed the Government Chemist, Sir Robert Robertson, declared that the tests carried out by Dr Henstock were themselves unreliable. The inadvertent result of all of this was, however, that a reliable test for tracing cannabis in tobacco mixtures was devised. By this test the offending cigarette brand, Ogden's 'St Julien', was cleared of suspicion. If there had been hashish in the Shrewsbury cigarette pouch, and there was now no clear evidence that there had been, then the Customs and Excise concluded that 'the presumption is that the hashish was mixed with the tobacco by the consumer after the tobacco had been sold in retail'.[15]

Meanwhile the original account of this story in the *British Medical Journal* had sparked an excited exchange of letters in subsequent issues. Lieutenant-Colonel W. S. J. Shaw of the Indian Medical Service wrote with his observations on 'Cannabis Indica: A "Dangerous Drug"'. He maintained that it was strange that cannabis indica and the various preparations made from the substance had not been included in the Dangerous Drugs Act. After acknowledging the recent flurry of newspaper attention on the subject, he became the latest in a long line to trot out the oft-disputed[16] asylum statistics of Asia in pointing out 'in 17 to 20 per cent of male admissions to the Indian mental hospitals and asylums the insanity is directly traceable to Indian hemp . . . the insane habitual consumer almost always exhibits maniacal-depressive symptoms tending rapidly to dementia'. Aware of the interest in the subject closer to home, he offered the following examples of the relationship between cannabis use, insanity, vagrancy, and vice in Europeans.

In twenty-four years experience in India I have seen only three cases of the use of the drug as a 'dope' by Europeans. One of these was a well to do globe trotter who had taken drugs all his life and who had no particular interest in Indian hemp except to obtain prolongation of time. Another was an excise inspector who when we first met was compelled to turn his back, stoop, and view me from between his

---

[15] PRO HO 144/6073 Tobacco, Adulteration with Hashish 8 Feb. 1924.
[16] See Chapters 4 and 5.

legs in order to see me in the standing position. His insanity was caused by ganja and he recovered rapidly. The third was an habitual of the beachcomber type who had become demented.[17]

This set off a correspondence that was at first dominated by stories from the colonies. T. F. Hugh-Smith related stories of Asian mountain tribes and tobacco use and observed that 'the Afghans do not confine themselves to the soothing weed, but mix it up with a number of intoxicating and injurious substances, such as Indian hemp or charas'.[18] In similarly exotic vein E. Griffith-Jones wrote from the Public Health Laboratories in Cairo to observe that

I do not recollect having heard any previous case of such adulteration in England. In Egypt, and the East generally, as is well known, 'hashish' is mixed with tobacco—chiefly cigarette tobacco—with the deliberate intention of catering for the palate of the 'hashash'. Tobaccos and cigarettes admixed with hashish are expensive and can only be purchased clandestinely. The precise object of mixing cannabis indica with tobacco for sale in England is not clear.[19]

W. E. Dixon finally felt compelled to write something positive about cannabis. Now established as a Reader in Pharmacology at Cambridge and destined to serve on the Rolleston Committee on Morphine and Heroin Addiction in 1925, he had worked with cannabis as a young researcher at Cambridge in the 1890s and had published his conclusion that 'I believe it to be an exceedingly useful therapeutic agent' in the *British Medical Journal*.[20] Almost a quarter of a century afterwards he vigorously asserted that cannabis had no place alongside cocaine and morphine in the British legal system. 'The Ministry of Health to my mind were right not to include hemp in the Dangerous Drugs Act since to do so is but to call attention to a drug which from the nature of things it is impossible to use as a drug of addiction in this country, and the action of which, except to a few experts, is unknown here,' he argued, adding that 'I do not believe that active cannabis indica in a form suitable for smoking can be obtained in this country.'[21]

Dixon seems, however, to have been an isolated voice. Overall, cannabis was increasingly caught up in a web of concern spun out of little more than

---

[17] W. S. J. Shaw, 'Cannabis Indica: A "Dangerous Drug"', *British Medical Journal*, 2 (1923), 586.

[18] T. F. Hugh-Smith, 'Cannabis Indica in Smoking Tobacco', ibid. 590.

[19] Ibid. 1006.

[20] W. E. Dixon, 'The Pharmacology of Cannabis Indica', *British Medical Journal*, 2 (1899), 1356. See Chapter 6 of this book for more on Dixon's work with cannabis.

[21] W. E. Dixon, 'Smoking of Indian Hemp and Opium', *British Medical Journal*, 2 (1923), 1179.

aspersions and inferences. The press had excited itself about a hashish seizure in London that in fact proved only that immigrant communities in Britain possessed cannabis. This was certainly not illegal and indeed was not considered undesirable by the Home Office expert on drugs Sir Malcolm Delevingne, who had concluded that the market for the drug was largely that of Asian and Arabian sailors passing through the country's ports. The South Shields seizure very much bore out his observation and proved little more than the fact that the British police could not tell the difference between opium and a range of other drugs. The case of the Shrewsbury tobacco pouch showed only that the science of the period was relatively ineffective in detecting cannabis. However, the press did not dwell on these aspects of the cases that it had been reporting. Instead, newspaper accounts and medical journals embroiled cannabis products in tales that contained exotic foreigners, smuggling and the police, cigarettes adulterated with poisons, and helpless young provincial girls. Statements such as 'the continued smoking of even minute quantities of "hashish" is likely to prove exceedingly harmful' and allegations of 'a serious growth in the traffic of hashish, a deadly Eastern drug which induces madness, in this country' had been made and remained uncorrected or unchallenged in the popular press despite their lack of foundation.

As such it is no surprise that the subject was raised in Parliament. On Thursday 21 February 1924 James Gilbert's written question was answered in the House of Commons. The MP for Southwark Central, who had travelled in India and Burma and so may have encountered cannabis substances outside the UK, had asked the Secretary of State for the Home Department, 'whether, seeing that hashish is not included on the list of dangerous drugs which are under restriction of importation into this country, he has any information of the use of this drug in certain seaport towns; and whether he proposes to take any steps to add this drug to the list of dangerous drugs and under the same restrictions as apply to them'.[22] The Home Office was equal to the task and answered reassuringly.

I have no information to show that indulgence in the use of hashish is anything but rare in this country though it is possible it is practised to a certain extent among Oriental seamen visiting our ports. Hashish is not one of the drugs to which the International Opium Convention of 1912 applies though the Hague Conference recommended that its use be investigated. Any proposal for the extension to hashish of the restrictions relating to the drugs included in the Convention would have to be considered from the international standpoint and I understand

---

[22] *Hansard*, 169 (Fifth Series), 2028–9, 21 Feb. 1924.

that the League of Nations which by the Treaties of Peace is entrusted with the general supervision over the traffic in dangerous drugs, has not yet considered the question. The question is one in which other countries are more closely concerned than this country, but the position is being watched by my Department and if it appears desirable steps will be taken to raise the question before the Opium Advisory Committee of the League.

In putting this case the Under-Secretary of State, Rhys Davies, was simply echoing the conclusions of Malcolm Delevingne, who had scrawled a set of notes in response to the parliamentary question. After reviewing the South Shields seizure he was firmly of the opinion that 'the existing situation in this country does not at present call for the inclusion of hashish in the Dangerous Drugs Act'.[23] It is important to note then that while police, press, and parliament were viewing cannabis through a lens clouded by ideas about opium and cocaine, those who did know what they were talking about and who had all the facts to hand were not inclined to legislate on the issue of cannabis. W. E. Dixon, one of the few men to have closely observed experiments with cannabis and a Professor of Pharmacology at Cambridge, and Sir Malcolm Delevingne of the Home Office, the chief civil servant of the period to deal with the issue of drugs, both felt that cannabis had no place in existing regulations. However, privately civil servants admitted that they were aware of the pressure on them to act on hashish, one official acknowledging on 7 May 1924 that 'the Home Office is constantly being urged to place the drug "hashish" or Indian hemp within the provisions of the Dangerous Drugs Acts which at present are confined to the drugs of the International Opium Convention namely, opium, morphine, heroin and cocaine'.[24]

THE PHARMACEUTICAL SOCIETY, POISONS, AND CORN PLASTERS

In the end, however, it was not the Home Office that took the first steps towards imposing regulations on cannabis drugs. By the middle of 1924 cannabis was finally included in the Poisons Schedule. The *Pharmaceutical Journal* announced on 9 August 1924 that 'the proposed addition of cannabis and its resins is an outcome of cases that have come before the police

[23] PRO HO 144/6073 Hashish: Inclusion in the Dangerous Drugs Act 20 Feb. 1924.
[24] PRO HO 144/6073 Dagga or Indian Hemp 2 May 1924.

courts of the use of hashish and other narcotic preparations of cannabis'.[25] It was the Pharmaceutical Society that was responsible for deciding what was and what was not to be classified as a poison. A substance was officially recognized as poisonous when the Society recommended it as a new entry on the lists known as the Poisons Schedules. While amendments to the Dangerous Drugs Act went through Parliament the recommendations for inclusion on the Poisons List were simply rubber-stamped by the Privy Council. Cannabis received its stamp that same month and the only explanation given of this decision was that vague reference to 'cases that have come before the police courts'. As the only such case that can be traced is that already discussed, of Thomas Garza and Idris Abdullah, it seems that police bungling and media excitement had combined to panic the Pharmaceutical Society into finding cannabis a place on the Poisons Schedule despite the opposition to regulations by policy-makers at the Home Office and by drugs experts like Professor Dixon at Cambridge University.

There was a controversy in the House of Commons about this sudden classification of cannabis as a poison. However, this was not a matter of defending a medicine or a drug against regulation by a state. Rather, it was caused by confusion over the humble corn plaster. The first volley in this brief political skirmish was fired on the 2 April 1925 in the House of Commons when 'Mr Forrest asked the Home Sec whether he is aware that in consequence of the scheduling of cannabis indica as a poison all forms using it even for minor manufactures of a non-deleterious nature have had only from 26th February to 3rd April to label millions of articles and whether, in view of the impossibility of conforming within this time with the Regulations, he will postpone the date of their enforcement and in the meantime investigate the need for their existence in these specific cases'. This question was quickly followed by a similar one that narrowed the issue further: 'Mr Wormesley asked the Home Sec if he is aware that the Order of the Privy Council making cannabis indica a poison and which comes into force on 3rd April will inflict hardship on many small shopkeepers who are not members of the Pharmaceutical Society who stock articles such as corn plasters containing a small quantity of cannabis indica and will he postpone putting into operation the Order for one month to allow them to dispose of their stocks?' The Minister of Health, Sir W. Joynson-Hicks, stood to make it clear that 'there is no power to

[25] 'Proposed Additions to the Poison Schedule', *Pharmaceutical Journal*, 113 (1924), 194.

postpone the operation of this order'. He also pointed out that it was due to come into operation the following day and that there had been plenty of warning of the Order.

Under the Statute the resolution of the Council of the Pharmaceutical Society for the inclusion of a substance in the Poisons Schedule takes effect one month after the order of the Privy Council Office approving it has been advertised in the 'London Gazette'. As the resolution was passed as long ago as last August ample notice has been given to all interested parties; and there do not appear to be any grounds on which the Government could properly intervene now. I am sure that no harsh measures will be taken by the Pharmaceutical Society in the enforcement of the law.[26]

The debate, of course, was about the range of products of the period that contained elements of the cannabis plant for a variety of purposes and the effort involved in labelling these as poisons to conform with the new classification. The corn plaster, mentioned by Mr Wormesley, was already a particularly difficult issue before it entered the House of Commons. A representative of Taylor's Drug Company in Leeds had written to the Pharmaceutical Society's own journal in March of 1925 to ask, 'can anyone tell me a chemical test as to whether a corn paint or plaster contains the resins of cannabis sativa in an active state and not inert; also what is one to state on the poison label next January—the proportion of herb or extract or resins?'[27] The same man, the Chemist Director of the company, wrote again a week later. He pointed out that some firms had not used cannabis in corn preparations for over a decade and those that did boiled extract of cannabis with chlorophyll and alcohol before adding the mixture to their corn preparations. How was the chemist to begin working out how much cannabis was in that corn plaster, he wondered. In the same issue of the journal a former lecturer on Materia Medica at Guy's Hospital wrote to say that he could not work out why cannabis was in corn treatments in the first place as he was not sure that it had any anodyne effects.

As the public have become accustomed to the green colour of salicylic plasters and paint it is, of course, as well to retain the green colour but we do not want to be quacks and ascribe properties to our preparations which they do not possess.[28]

A trawl through records of the Pharmaceutical Society was the next step in this growing controversy and on 25 April an article from the 1883

[26] *Hansard*, 182 (Fifth Series), 1496, 2 Apr. 1925.
[27] 'Letters to the Editor', *Pharmaceutical Journal*, 114 (1925), 416.
[28] 'Cannabis Indica in Corn Plasters and Solvents', *Pharmaceutical Journal*, 114 (1925), 457.

volume of the journal was reproduced that asserted that cannabis was indeed in the corn paste as an anodyne.[29] However, the confusion took on an international dimension as the American Medical Association wrote to argue that 'the cannabis can play no role beyond that of a colouring agent'.[30] Indeed, the corn plaster even became a matter of international diplomacy at the Opium Conference early in 1925, although the evidence suggests that the matter was not taken quite as seriously in Geneva as it had been in London. Sir Malcolm Delevingne reported, with a slyly wry tone, the proposal regarding cannabis medicines in the Convention by noting that 'it only applies to the extract and tincture and not to preparations of which the extract or tincture forms part. It would not apply therefore to the corn plaster of which we have heard so much.'[31]

The fact remains however that in a decade when cannabis found itself declared a poison and in which it became subject to international laws on drugs, the corn plaster controversy provides the only serious discussion among legislators about the regulation of Indian hemp substances. There were no objections to cannabis itself being placed on the Poisons Schedule and being subjected to the Poisons Laws. As for the Opium Convention and its stipulations on cannabis the records note that they were put together in a Bill and when presented to Parliament this was simply 'passed without amendment' in 1925.[32] The errors of the police, the excitability of the press, the panic of the pharmacists, and the indifference of Parliament meant that cannabis passed into law and was subject to regulation, despite the opinions of the experts, because of little more than innuendo and suspicion and without anything approaching a well-informed debate.

[29] 'Cannabis Indica in Corn Solvents', ibid. 468.
[30] Ibid. 645.
[31] PRO HO 144/6073 Hashish Compromise 14 Feb. 1925.
[32] *General Index of the Journals of the House of Commons from 1921–1930* (HMSO Press, London, 1931), 107.

9

Conclusion: Cannabis and British Government, 1800–1928

Three sets of conclusions may be drawn from this study. The first relates to patterns of use of cannabis. The second is more speculative and regards the usefulness for current debates of the information that British administrators, officials, and observers generated about cannabis in their dealings with it before 1928. The third is perhaps the most important and focuses on the circumstances in which cannabis policy and cannabis laws have been formulated.

As regards consumption of cannabis, it is clear that there was very little use of preparations of the plant in the UK in the period 1800–1928. British doctors reported using it infrequently to control pain, swelling, and spasms and the only habitual recreational consumers of the drug in this country were visitors from Asia and Africa who were usually passing through as sailors or itinerant workers. However, this did not mean that the British had no experience of societies where preparations of Indian hemp were common and popular. It was in the empire that British administrators, doctors, and scientists encountered populations and cultures where cannabis substances were resorted to extensively and for a variety of purposes, as medicines, as tonics, and as intoxicants. By the 1920s a range of individuals and various departments of colonial states across the globe had been collecting data on cannabis and the consumption of the preparations of the plant for over a century and much of this data had been fed back into metropolitan government and scientific circles throughout the period.

Perhaps just as important as these observations on the origins of this data is the nature of the information that the British gathered on the drug. The first point worth noting is that British doctors and scientists consistently acknowledged the potential of cannabis as a medicine for a range of complaints and conditions. William O'Shaughnessy back in the 1840s in Calcutta for example concluded after experiments with cannabis in cases of tetanus that 'to me they seem unequivocally to shew, that when given boldly, and in large doses, the resin of Hemp is capable of arresting effectually the progress of this formidable disease, and in a large proportion of cases of effecting a perfect cure'.[1] J. Russell Reynolds, Physician to Queen Victoria's household, was in full agreement with these arguments over fifty years after the Calcutta experiments, stating that 'Indian hemp when pure and administered carefully is one of the most valuable medicines we possess'. The Indian Hemp Drugs Commission was sure that 'cannabis indica must be looked upon as one of the most important drugs of Indian Materia Medica'. It went on to note that it was frequently used in various forms in India to treat dysentery, to ward off malaria, to calm piles, to soothe inflammation, and as a local anaesthetic. It was also useful for stimulating appetite and digestion and for giving 'staying power' to 'gymnasts, wrestlers and musicians, palki-bearers and porters, divers and postal runners . . . on occasions of especially severe exertion'.[2] W. E. Dixon, who was to go on to serve on the Rolleston Committee in the 1920s that was to lay the foundations of British approach to drug abuse for much of the rest of the century, was similarly keen to argue of cannabis that 'I believe it to be an exceedingly useful therapeutic agent, one not likely to lead to abuse and producing in proper dosage no untoward after-effects'.[3] Overall then, British doctors and scientists have known for 200 years what the BMA stated as recently as 1997, that is that cannabinoids 'have a therapeutic potential in a number of medical conditions in which present drugs or other treatments are not fully adequate'.[4] Much like their predecessors the doctors that wrote this BMA report were keen to see cannabinoids used in the treatment of 'intractable pain'.

Importantly, however, British doctors and scientists regularly reported the side effects of using cannabis based medicines. O'Shaughnessy observed

[1] W. B. O'Shaughnessy, 'On the Preparations of Indian Hemp', in *Transactions of the Medical and Physical Society of Bengal* (1838–40), 461.

[2] *Report of the Indian Hemp Drugs Commission 1893–4* (Simla, 1894), i. 174–82.

[3] W. E. Dixon, 'The Pharmacology of Cannabis Indica' *British Medical Journal*, 2 (1899), 1356.

[4] British Medical Association, *Therapeutic Uses of Cannabis* (Harwood Academic Publishers, Amsterdam, 1997), 78.

that on administering cannabis drugs to his students 'after an average interval of one hour, the pulse was increased in fulness and frequency; the surface of the body glowed; the appetite became extraordinary; vivid ideas crowded the mind; unusual loquacity occurred; and with scarcely any exception, great aphrodisia was experienced'. The Report of the Indian Hemp Drugs Commission noted that side effects could vary widely so that sometimes there was 'exhilaration and slightly dizzy sensation', sometimes 'the man becomes peevish, stupefied, sees double; and occasionally it may cause vomiting', then again it seemed that 'conjunctiva become suffused and red, and the moisture dries in the throat and lips'. Dr Bovill, serving in India, noted the psychological side effects of a large dose of ganja that he had smoked by way of experiment.[5]

The smoke of 5 and 6 grains inhaled into the lungs caused singing in the ears, feeling of heat and oppression in cardiac region, rapid pulse, and at intervals a feeling of apprehension of danger. Visions of all kinds float before the eyes, changing rapidly, of bright or sparkling appearance . . . the inhalation of 10 grains produced the same symptoms in more marked form, with decided hallucinations of hearing voices, bells, railway whistles, some unsteadiness of hand and gait, forcible vomiting without any feeling of nausea.

He decided after such an experience that 'this sensation is decidedly very disagreeable, not such as to encourage the repetition of the experiment'. Again, these observations very much anticipated recent medical conclusions on the subject. The BMA report of 1997 listed sedation, euphoria, hallucinations, paranoia, and impaired memory as the psychological results of using cannabis and cannabinoids in clinical practice. Physical side effects that they noted included blurred vision, coughing and chest discomfort, slurred speech, and ataxia (poor balance).

Opinions were divided on the psychological impact of this social use of the drugs. Lunatic asylums in India and Egypt churned out statistics that were used as scientific evidence of a connection between cannabis use and mental health problems. However, there was a number of problems with these statistics. Those compiling them doubted their accuracy, Surgeon-Major Cobb noting for example that 'in the Dacca Asylum there are at present 53 out of 240 lunatics whose insanity has been attributed to ganja. In many of these cases the fact of their being ganja smokers is doubtful.' Indeed, he was at pains to stress that even were these numbers correct then in the context of all the users of the drug in local society 'the proportion of insanes whose insanity can be attributed to hemp to the large number of users of the

[5] Evidence of Surgeon Lieutenant Colonel E. Bovill, in *Report of the IHDC 1893–4*, iv. 283.

drug is almost infinitesimally small'.[6] Some, however, preferred to abandon the evidence altogether and to assert that cannabis drugs must produce mental illness simply because of their properties: 'it appears that alcohol, opium, chloral and perhaps some other stimulants and narcotics cause insanity and there is no reason why Indian hemp should not do so too'.[7]

Others still were sure that use of cannabis did not cause insanity, but rather acted to stimulate a mental illness that was already lurking in the mind of the individual: 'my general impression is that ganja is an exciting cause of insanity, as alcohol is. Probably in most cases there is a weak brain, which the ganja acted on, or a tendency to insanity.'[8] For Surgeon Captain Charles MacTaggart use of ganja was not a cause of mental illness, it was evidence of an already established psychological problem: 'no doubt in many cases of insanity supposed to be due to ganja, the ganja smoking is a symptom of the disease and not the cause'.[9] However, a colleague differed on this as he thought that cannabis was used by those already afflicted with mental illness in order to alleviate its distressing effects —'I certainly think that the drugs are sometimes resorted to by persons suffering with mental anxiety or brain disease to obtain relief (just as Europeans often resort to alcohol with that object)'.[10] Surgeon Lieutenant Colonel O'Brien was, however, altogether convinced that 'in regard to insanity, I have long thought that the moderate use of hemp drugs does not produce insanity but that it prevents it. I have for many years believed that the moderate use of hemp and opium is one of the reasons that there is so little insanity in this country.'[11] There were even those in the nineteenth century that used cannabis to treat insanity, and indeed Thomas Clouston won the Fothergillian Gold Medal of the Medical Society of London in 1870 for his work with hemp drugs in the treatment of mental illness at the hospital that he was in charge of in Carlisle.

Opinion on the matter of whether cannabis use caused insanity was as divided among medical observers before 1928 as it is among scientists and campaigners on the issue today. Part of the reason for this was the differentiation made by many investigators and observers between 'moderate' and 'excessive' users. John Warnock in Cairo conceded that 'probably only excessive users ... become so insane as to need asylum treatment. Whether

[6] Evidence of Surgeon Major R. Cobb, in ibid., iii. 291.
[7] Evidence of Surgeon Lieutenant Colonel E. Bovill, ibid., iv. 285.
[8] Evidence of Surgeon Lieutenant Colonel W. Flood Murray, ibid., iii. 264.
[9] Evidence of Surgeon Captain C. MacTaggart, ibid., v. 123.
[10] Evidence of Surgeon Lieutenant Colonel W. R. Hooper, ibid. 111.
[11] Evidence of Surgeon Lieutenant Colonel B. O'Brien, ibid. 121.

the moderate use of hasheesh has ill effects I have no means of judging.'[12]
Surgeon Lieutenant Colonel J. McConaghey, the Civil Surgeon of
Allahabad, was fairly typical in arguing to the IHDC that 'if used for a
prolongued period in excess these drugs are injurious; they blunt the moral
senses, impair the physical powers, pervert the brain functions and deaden
the intellect'. In answer to the question 'does the habitual moderate use of
any of these drugs produce any noxious effects?' he answered clearly, 'if
moderation is strictly adhered to, no'. Others embellished this answer,
Surgeon Lieutenant Colonel G. C. Hall stating, 'I believe the moderate
use of these drugs to be harmless; my reason for my answer being that I have
seen many moderate consumers who had taken these drugs for years and not
suffered in health in any way.'[13] This contrasted starkly with the excessive
user described by Dr McConaghy in Pune, 'the habitual excessive use of
bhang or ganja impairs the constitution, injures digestion, causes loss
of appetite and bronchitis, impairs the moral sense and induces laziness. It
may deaden the intellect and produce insanity, especially in those predis-
posed to nervous affections.'[14] However, nowhere was the definition of
moderation satisfactorily arrived at, and Dr MacNamara in Assam confessed that 'I can't define moderation no more [*sic*] than I can in the case
of alcohol. The limit is reached when any ill effects are apparent, when the
limit is crossed.'[15]

As for the physical impact of regular use of the drug there was also
division among British observers. An observer in Nellore argued that 'habitual use tends to impair consitution by producing loss of appetite and
emaciation and a constant irritable cough'[16] and a colleague further south
in Vizagapatam conjured up the image of 'the habitual excessive consumer
[who] is dull, dirty and ill-clad; the eyes protrude, cheek bones prominent,
the body thin and emaciated, with a pale sallow complexion'.[17] On the
other hand there were those who were adamant that 'I have known men
in good health and in full exercise of mental and physical faculties who
have so used ganja for from fourteen to sixteen years'[18] or who were sure
that 'during my twenty years' attendance at dispensaries in these provinces . . . I have had no experience in the treatment of illnesses caused by

---

[12] J. Warnock, 'Insanity from Hasheesh', *Journal of Mental Science*, 49 (1903), 109.
[13] Evidence of Surgeon Lieutenant Colonel G. C. Hall, in *Report of the IHDC 1893–4*, v. 117.
[14] Evidence of Surgeon Lieutenant W. McConaghy, ibid., vii. 142.
[15] Evidence of Surgeon Major J. MacNamara, ibid., iv. 553.
[16] Evidence of Surgeon Major W. F. Thomas, ibid., vi. 288.
[17] Evidence of Apothecary N. H. Daniel, ibid. 299.
[18] Evidence of Surgeon Lieutenant Colonel E.G. Russell, ibid., iv. 274.

ganja, charas or bhang. I do not believe that such exist.'[19] Some went even further to provide evidence that cannabis did no physical harm to the user, Surgeon Captain J. H. Tull Walsh reporting that after cutting up the body of a deceased consumer, 'as regards the general appearance of the various organs of the body, and especially with regard to coarse lesions of the brain, these cases show nothing which could be ascribed to the action of ganja'.[20] Indeed, the IHDC itself was convinced that the use of cannabis products could actually have beneficial physical effects and it quoted Dr Edward Smith approvingly as he concluded of cannabis that 'it increases the assimilation of food both of the flesh and heat forming kind, and with abundance of food must promote nutrition'.[21]

On the issue of whether cannabis was a gateway drug that was likely to lead to consumers developing a craving for other psycho-active substances and experiences, most British observers seemed uninterested in the subject. Indeed, the only time that cannabis users seemed likely to turn to other substances was when their access to the drug was restricted by considerations of price. In the 1870s the Board of Revenue in Bengal noted sourly that 'ganja has been getting dearer and dearer of late years and it may fairly be presumed that even if there were no ganja to be had, a certain proportion of the population would go mad from the abuse of some other drug. A prohibition... against the use of ganja in any shape would be difficult to enforce and if the prohibition were successfully enforced, some other drug would probably take the place of ganja.'[22] Two decades later the IHDC could conclude that 'hemp drug revenue has risen when the price of liquor has been raised and that it has fallen when under the establishment of the outstill instead of the central distillery system liquor has been made more plentiful and more cheap'.[23]

As for the social impact of cannabis use, there were similarly opposing views. In Bengal it seemed that most agreed with the Inspector-General of Police that 'there is no established connection between hemp drugs and professional crime'.[24] However, across in Allahabad the Superintendent of Police believed that 'excessive use... promotes poverty and despair and all the results of a debased life which naturally must lead to a criminal life'.[25]

---

[19] Evidence of Surgeon Lieutenant Colonel B. O'Brien, ibid., v. 120.
[20] Evidence of Surgeon Captain J. H. Tull Walsh, ibid., iv. 301.
[21] *Report of the IHDC 1893–4*, i. 181.
[22] 'Papers Relating to the Consumption of Ganja and Other Drugs in India', *British Parliamentary Papers*, 66 (Hansard, London, 1891), 66.
[23] *Report of the IHDC 1893–4*, i. 137.
[24] Evidence of R. Henry, ibid., iv. 235.
[25] Evidence of Mr L. H. Lovett-Thomas to IHDC, ibid., v. 109.

John Warnock, speaking of his observations in Egypt, was also sure that there was a link arguing that 'I find that persons insane from hasheesh have a proneness to commit crimes, especially those of violence, and I have a strong suspicion that much disorderly conduct results from hasheesh smoking just as alcohol among Europeans leads to such misconduct'.[26] Others pointed out, however, that 'the only connection between these drugs and crime that I know of is that when a man has made up his mind to a crime, and has not the pluck to do it, he takes the drug to give him Dutch courage'.[27] However, it was feared by some that sudden violence could be the outcome of a particularly enthusiastic debauch in cannabis substances: 'excessive indulgence in ganja incites a man to unpremeditated crime, the effects of rashness and violence of temper caused by smoking it,'[28] argued the District Superintendent of Police in Dinajpur. Of the 600 witnesses that commented on the relationship between cannabis use and violent crime to the IHDC, however, it reported that two-thirds denied that there was such a link and it concluded that 'occasionally, but apparently very rarely indeed, excessive indulgence in hemp drugs may lead to violent crime'.[29]

However, the one crime that they did agree on was smuggling. It was noted that 'the smuggling of ganja from the Tributary States of Orissa into British territory has a long history'[30] and that in Burma, where the British had tried to prevent cannabis use among the local population since the 1870s, officials were forced to admit that 'I am afraid, I must say, that the prohibition is ineffective in Rangoon. The consumers get their ganja all the same and hundreds are getting a living by it. I do not believe that ganja could be stopped even by an army of officials and constant interference with the people.'[31] Much the same story was told in Egypt, and within ten years of asserting their administration in the country British officials could write that 'the main facts of the case are very simple. On the one hand the importation and use of haschisch is forbidden by law. On the other hand, it is notorious that the drug is largely imported and very generally used. It would, under any circumstances, be very difficult to stop haschisch being smuggled into the country.'[32]

---

[26] Warnock, 'Insanity from Hasheesh', 110.

[27] Evidence of Mr F. Porter in *Report of the IHDC*, v. 108.

[28] Evidence of Mr F. H. Tucker, Ibid. 241.

[29] *Report of the IHDC*, i. 264.

[30] Ibid. 314.   [31] Ibid. 340.

[32] Reports from Her Majesty's Representatives in Egypt, Greece and Turkey on Regulations Affecting the Importation and Sale of Haschisch, *Parliamentary Papers*, 89 (1893–4), 294.

Finally, opinion also seems split on whether cannabis users were lazy and disinclined to work. There was a constant stream of complaints that this was the case. For example, in South Africa allegations by white employers about the effect of cannabis on the local population of migrant workers led the Indian Immigrants Commission to conclude that 'it renders the Indian Immigrant unfit and unable to perform, with satisfaction to the employer, that work for which he was specially brought to the Colony'.[33] In Egypt Warnock reckoned that the 'cannabinomaniac' was 'a good for nothing, lazy fellow, who lives by begging and stealing and pesters his relations for money to buy hasheesh'.[34] However, there were also those that were sure that the drugs were central to a good day's work for manual labourers: 'persons whose employment subjects them to great exertions and fatigues, such as palki-bearers etc. are solely enabled to perform the wonderful feats they not unfrequently do by being supported and rendered insensible to fatigue by ganja'.[35] Surgeon Lieutenant Colonel E. Bovill, the Civil Surgeon at Patna in 1894, was convinced that 'I do not know of any case in which a previously energetic person has become lazy and immoral through the use of hemp drugs'.[36] The IHDC reported that 'all classes of labourers, especially such as blacksmiths, miners, and coolies, are said more or less generally to use the drugs as a rule in moderation to alleviate fatigue'.[37]

When viewed broadly then it seems that there is one basic conclusion that can be drawn from a survey of the attitudes towards cannabis products that developed among the range of British doctors, scientists, policemen, administrators, and taxmen that recorded their experiences of those substances and of societies where they were commonly used as medicines, tonics, and intoxicants. The conclusion is that there is no conclusion, that there is no generally held or widely applicable statement that can be made from all of these observations, trials, and assertions on any of the various issues of cannabis and health or cannabis and society. The scientific, political, and governmental statements on cannabis came no nearer to a consensus on cannabis in the nineteenth and early twentieth centuries than they have at the end of the twentieth and at the start of the twenty-first centuries.

[33] *Report of the Indian Immigrants Commission (Natal Legislative Council) 1885–87* (Davis, Pietermaritzburg, 1887), 7.
[34] Warnock, 'Insanity from Hasheesh', 103.
[35] 'Papers Relating to the Consumption of Ganja and Other Drugs in India', 11.
[36] The quotes from the IHDC are taken from interviews with medical officers across India. See *Report of the IHDC 1893–4*, iv. 262–308, 549–560; v. 110–36; vi. 274–99; vii. 135–52.
[37] Ibid., i. 182.

This, however, is perhaps the most important conclusion that can be drawn from past experience for current debates about cannabis. Cannabis and cannabis preparations are complex substances that can have a variety of impacts in the short and long terms which are ameliorated by such factors as the physiology of the individual and his or her general state of health, the diet and other intakes of the user, the potency of the preparations taken, the mood and mental health of the consumer, and the social context of consumption. Yet these facts alone rarely determine the attitudes formed by individuals and the policies decided upon by governments when considering the subject. In explaining the lack of consensus and in seeking to analyse the reasons why individuals and administrations came to the conclusions that they did, this study has begun to show that attitudes towards substances like cannabis are formed in the context of vested interests, moral judgements, and political agendas. Ainslie was a teetotaller and a moralizing Christian who viewed all intoxication as sinful. O'Shaughnessy was an ambitious man who was advocating cannabis as a medicine in a period when there was a growing market for 'wonder-drugs' in Europe and a curiosity among the more adventurous of his colleagues in India about the possibilities of Asian therapies and substances. The asylum statistics that convinced many of the link between cannabis use and mental illness were compiled by British doctors in India who were driven by a need to fill in the forms and who were mystified by much of the behaviour of the locals because of their profound ignorance of the societies they governed. William Caine was eager to portray cannabis as an evil once he had discovered that the colonial government that was his stated foe derived a revenue from the sale of the drug. The Indian Hemp Drugs Commission was dominated by Government of India officials who were aware of the usefulness of the revenue from cannabis to the administration that employed them. The Egyptian delegates at the League of Nations Opium Convention were conscious of the embarrassment that they could cause to their colonial oppressors through the issue of cannabis. The reporters back in London knew from experience that drugs scandals made good copy and as such were only too happy to portray cannabis as the new foreign intoxicant about to sweep a decadent West End.

Finally, and before considering the third set of conclusions about policy, it is worth summarizing the story of how cannabis first became a matter for restrictions and regulations in Britain. The Home Office had carefully monitored stories about cannabis use in the UK throughout the 1920s and saw no reason for the drugs to be included in the Dangerous Drugs Acts. Indeed Sir Malcolm Delevingne, the chief policy-maker on drugs of the period at the Home Office, was engaged in fighting off attempts to include Indian hemp substances in the international laws that were evolving in negotiations at the Second Opium Convention. Medical opinion on cannabis was divided and commonly ill-informed. Few devoted much time to the subject, but it is interesting that those that could claim to have actually followed debates about drugs in general and about cannabis in particular over a whole career, men like Professor W. E. Dixon, a Reader in Pharmacy at Cambridge, were adamant that Indian hemp had no place alongside opium and cocaine in the regulatory system of the UK.

Despite this 'expert' opinion of civil servants and scientists, and despite the fact that there really was no domestic cannabis use in the 1920s, the drug did enter the statute books in that decade through two routes. The first was via Geneva and the Second Opium Conference. As was seen in Chapter 7, this was the result of an impassioned campaign by the Egyptian delegate founded on scanty and highly questionable medical data that was supplied by a British colonial doctor. This campaign suc-ceeded because of the indifference of most other delegates at the meeting and because cannabis became enmeshed in the complex politics of the opium debate.

The second route into law was via the Pharmaceutical Society and its power to identify substances to be listed under the Poisons Act. The only reason given for nominating cannabis in 1924 was that it had come to the Society's attention because it had noticed 'cases that have come before the police courts of the use of hashish'. The previous chapter has shown that the police were unable to identify cannabis accurately, that they wrongly thought it to be similar in its properties to opium, and that it was only encountered by the authorities when policing immigrant communities. It also showed that such a case was briefly but energetically reported by the media in a flurry of stories that recreated the drug scares of the war period that had been focused on cocaine and opiates. These stories represented cannabis quite falsely as a new plague about to sweep London that was directly comparable to heroin and cocaine and would induce insanity. Police confusion and media hype nevertheless seem to have impressed the pharmacists, who acted quickly on cannabis, apparently without consulting the Home Office or indeed experts within their own ranks. This then is the reason that the history of cannabis and British government before 1928 is important. It demonstrates that assessments of drugs, and indeed laws and regulations that control medicinal and intoxicating substances, have been formed on the basis of political and moral agendas and reactions rather than on informed debate or well-established policy models.

Indeed, this impression is confirmed as the broader sweep of the experiences of British government of cannabis products is considered. In India, colonial officials began to associate cannabis with criminality at about the same time that they began trying to tax the trade in Indian hemp products more efficiently. Once a product becomes the subject of a state levy, and once the traditional producers and suppliers of that article act to protect their profits by evading that levy, that product and those traders become suspicious to administrators seeking to maximize the state's revenues. Cannabis assumed an air of illegality because the colonial state in India imposed duties on it and branded as criminal all who sought to preserve their income from trade in the substance by trying to dodge payment of those duties.

Similarly, British government in India produced statistics that seemed to prove a link between mental illness and cannabis use. These were widely used in the empire and beyond to cast a shadow over the use of cannabis. The statistics were discredited in the 1890s and indeed look highly questionable to this day, and are apparently based on poor sampling, administrative expedience, and the misjudgements of a complex society by ignorant or ill-informed colonizers. Yet the criticisms of the 1890s went largely unheard and these statistics, and other data churned out in similar circumstances, continued to be quoted authoritatively and to impact upon policy into the 1920s.

Of course there were those that were arguing the case for cannabis and who were sure that it was a useful medicine and a harmless intoxicant. These were often powerful and important officials and scientists in both metropolitan and colonial circles who produced evidence that was every bit as compelling as that cited by opponents of the drug. Yet the fact is that ultimately these voices were ignored and cannabis was increasingly associated with insanity, criminality, and with those other suspicious substances, cocaine and opium. This study has argued that the development of this distrust of the drug was due to political, moral, and cultural factors that often resulted in exaggerated, ill-founded, and downright mistaken perceptions. Nevertheless, despite these unsound foundations, these perceptions generated policies that kicked off the process of governing cannabis that continues to this day.

It is worth dwelling on the details of this last point. As was stated in the Introduction, the present government has consistently referred back with approval to the policies on cannabis of its predecessors. Indeed, until recently it based its position on the presupposition that its predecessors, specifically those drafting the 1971 Misuse of Drugs Act, got it right in their classification of cannabis. Yet when the reasoning of these predecessors back in the 1960s and 1970s is examined it is found that they also looked to precedent to bolster their stance in the belief that what had gone before must have been properly considered and established for rational reasons. In other words for over thirty years governments have been proceeding with attitudes towards and policies on cannabis based on the assumption that these attitudes and policies were well founded and rational. History was at the heart of policy.

Significantly, however, there seems never to have been a comprehensive attempt to check or to verify that these attitudes and policies were indeed well founded and rational. As such, the assumption made has been a blind one. This study has begun what, in such a light, looks to be a long overdue procedure of examining the history of government policy and of official attitudes in the UK by focusing on the processes that lead to the first instances of cannabis regulation in the 1920s. It has suggested that this history is one of shaky science, misjudgements and misunderstandings, media scares, and once-important but now long-dead political agendas.

Bibliography

OFFICIAL PUBLICATIONS AND RECORDS
(LISTED BY DATE)

UK Government

Hansard's Parliamentary Debates, 1876–1925.

Reports from Her Majesty's Representatives in Egypt, Greece and Turkey on Regulations Affecting the Importation and Sale of Haschisch, *Parliamentary Papers*, 89 (1893–4).

Correspondence Relative to the International Opium Commission at Shanghai 1909 (HMSO, London, 1909).

Report of the British Delegates to the International Opium Conference Held at the Hague, December 1911–January 1912 (HMSO, London, 1912).

General Index of the Journals of the House of Commons from 1921–1930 (HMSO, Press, London, 1931).

Standing Committee A, *Misuse of Drugs Bill*, 17 Nov. 1970.

Select Committee on Science and Technology 2nd Report 1998–9, *Cannabis: Government Response* (The Stationery Office, London, 1999).

Select Committee on Science and Technology, 2nd Report 2000–1, *Therapeutic Uses of Cannabis* (www.parliament.the-stationery-office.co.uk).

Public Record Office (PRO) CO 323/973/9 Drug smuggling: Activities of Henri de Monfried, 1927.

PRO CO 530/111 Mons. de Monfried, 1927.

PRO FO 841/146 Alexander Tanti for Permitting the Use and Smoking of Hashish, 1914.

PRO HO 45/24739 Committee on Draft Regulations for the Dangerous Drugs Act 1920: Signed Report, 1921.

PRO HO 144/6073 Dangerous Drugs and Poisons: Traffic in Indian Hemp, Hashish, etc., 1922–6.

PRO PC 8/803 Inter-Departmental Conference on Opium Traffic, 1916.

PRO WO 33/881 Minutes of the Proceedings of and Precis Prepared for the Army Council for the Years 1915 and 1916.

Colonial Government

Report of the Indian Immigrants Commission (Natal Legislative Council) 1885–87 (Davis, Pietermaritzburg, 1887).

The case notes of the Lucknow Lunatic Asylum (in the private collection of Dr Aditya Kumar of the Agra Mental Hospital).

India Office Library L/Mil/9/383/124 Assistant Surgeon's Papers.

Annual Reports on the Insane Asylums in Bengal for the Year (Calcutta, 1868–74).

Annual Report of the Lunatic Asylums in the Punjab for the Year 1871–72 (Lahore, 1873).

Report on the Lunatic Asylums in the Central Provinces for the Year 1880 (Nagpur, 1881).

Report of the Commission Appointed by the Government of Bengal to Enquire into the Excise of Country Spirit in Bengal 1883–84 (Bengal Secretariat Press, Calcutta, 1884).

Papers Regarding the Cultivation of Hemp in India (Agra Secundra Orphan Press, 1855).

'Papers Relating to the Consumption of Ganja and Other Drugs in India', *British Parliamentary Papers*, 66 (Hansard, London, 1891).

Prain, D., *Report on the Cultivation and use of Ganja* (Bengal Secretariat Press, Calcutta, 1893).

Report of the Indian Hemp Drugs Commission 1893–4 (Simla, 1894), vols. i–viii.

Memorandum on Excise Administration in India so far as it is concerned with Hemp Drugs (Government Printing Office, Simla, 1901–22).

Rainy, G., *Report on the Manufacture and Smuggling of Ganja* (Bengal Secretariat Press, Calcutta, 1904).

'The Report of the Committee Appointed to Enquire into Certain Aspects of Opium and Ganja Consumption', *Assam Gazette* (10 Dec. 1918).

Maharashtra State Archives Bombay General File 1913/100.

International Opium Conferences at Geneva, 1924–5: Report of the Indian Delegation, in Maharashtra State Archives 1926 File 5639/24C.

League of Nations

Report of the Advisory Committee on Traffic in Opium 1921.

Minutes of the Advisory Committee on Traffic in Opium and Other Dangerous Drugs, 1921–4.

Records of the Second Opium Conference, 1924–5.

ARTICLES AND PAPERS

(Listed in alphabetical order by author. Where article has no author identified it is listed in alphabetical order under the name of the journal that published it.)

Abkari   *Abkari: The Quarterly Organ of the Anglo-Indian Temperance Association*, 1892–1904

BMJ   *British Medical Journal*

EMJ   *Edinburgh Medical Journal*

JMS   *Journal of Mental Science*
PJ   *Pharmaceutical Journal*
PMSJ   *Provincial Medical and Surgical Journal*

'An ex-Commissioner of Bengal on Indian Hemp', *Abkari*, 13 (Apr. 1893).
'Annual Report 1892–3', *Abkari*, 14 (July 1893).
'Hemp Drugs', *Abkari*, 18 (1894).
'Hemp Drugs in Bengal', *Abkari*, 16 (1894).
'Hemp Drugs in North Africa', *Abkari*, 26 (1896).
'Indian Hemp from a Public Health Point of View', *Abkari*, 14 (1893).
'Notes on Ganja', *Abkari*, 13 (Apr. 1893).
BARROW, B., 'A Case of Dysmenorrhoea in which the Tincture of Cannabis Indica was Employed with some Observations upon that Drug', *PMSJ* (1847).
BATHO, R., 'Cannabis Indica', *BMJ* (1883).
BEDDOE, J., 'Cannabis Indica', *BMJ* (1883).
BERRIDGE, V., 'War Conditions and Narcotics Control: the passing of Defence of the Realm Act Regulation 40B', *Journal of Social Policy*, 7/3 (1978).
——'The Origins of the English Drug "Scene" 1890–1930', *Medical History*, 32 (1988).
BEVERIDGE, A., and RENVOIZE, E., 'Electricity: A History of its Use in the Treatment of Mental Illness in Britain during the Second Half of the Nineteenth Century', *British Journal of Psychiatry*, 153 (1988).
'India and the Colonies', *BMJ* (July–Dec. 1894).
'The Indian Hemp Drugs Commission', *BMJ* (Jan.–June 1895).
BROWN, J., 'Cannabis Indica: A Valuable Remedy in Menorrhagia', *BMJ* (1883).
CHATURVEDI, G., et al., 'Medicinal Use of Opium and Cannabis in Medieval India', *Indian Journal of History of Science*, 16/1 (1981).
CLOUSTON, T. S., 'Observations and Experiments on the Use of Opium, Bromide of Potassium and Cannabis Indica in Insanity, Especially in Regard to the Effects of the Two Latter Together', *British and Foreign Medico-Chirurgical Review*, 46 (1870) and 47 (1871).
——'The Cairo Asylum: Dr Warnock on Hasheesh Insanity', *JMS*, 42 (1896).
CORBYN, F., 'Management and Diseases of Infants under the Influence of the Climate of India', *Lancet*, 2 (1828/9).
CRONIN, J., 'Cannabis Indica', *BMJ* (1883).
DIXON, W. E., 'The Pharmacology of Cannabis Indica', *BMJ*, 2 (1899).
——'Smoking of Indian Hemp and Opium', *BMJ*, 2 (1923).
DOUGLAS, D., 'On the Use of Indian Hemp in Chorea', *EMJ*, 14 (1869).
DOWNER, R., 'Cannabis Indica in Smoking Tobacco', *BMJ*, 2 (1923).
'A Survey of Illegal Drugs', *The Economist*, 28 July 2001.
EVANS, T., 'The Cultivation of "Ganja" by the Indian Government', *Abkari*, 3 (1892).

FAYRER, J., 'A Case of Traumatic Tetanus Treated by Opium Smoking and Internal Administration of Chloroform and Hemp', *EMJ*, 10 (1865).

FOULIS, J., 'Two Cases of Poisoning by Cannabis Indica', *EMJ*, 8 (1900).

'Potted History' *Independent on Sunday*, 26 Dec. 1999.

HUGH-SMITH, T. F., 'Cannabis Indica in Smoking Tobacco', *BMJ*, 2 (1923).

IRELAND, W., 'On Thought without Words and the Relation of Words to Thought', *JMS*, 24 (1878).

JACKSON, T., 'Uncertain Action of Cannabis Indica', *BMJ* (1857).

'Cannabis Indica in Gastric Disorders', *Lancet*, 2 (1890).

'The Hemp Drugs Commission', *Lancet*, 1 (1895).

'Poisoning by Indian Hemp: Autopsy', *Lancet*, 2 (1880).

LEY, W., 'On the Efficacy of Indian Hemp in some Convulsive Disorders' *PMSJ*, 4 (1842).

MARSHALL, C., 'The Active Principle of Indian Hemp: A Preliminary Investigation' *Lancet*, 1 (1897).

——'A Review of Recent Work on Cannabis Indica', *PJ* 15 (1902).

——'Report on the Standardization of Preparations of Indian Hemp', *BMJ*, 1 (1911); *BMJ* 1 (1912).

MAUDSLEY, H., 'Insanity and its Treatment', *JMS*, 17 (1871–2).

MOON, J., 'Sir William Brooke O'Shaughnessy: The Foundations of Fluid Therapy and the Indian Telegraph Service', *New England Journal of Medicine*, 276 (1967).

OLIVER, J., 'On the Action of Cannabis Indica', *BMJ* (Jan.–June 1883).

'General Retrospect', *PMSJ* (1849).

'Insanity in Egypt', *PMSJ* (1846).

PEEL NESBITT, W., 'Cannabis Indica', *BMJ* (1883).

'Cannabinol', *PJ*, 7 (1898–9).

'Cannabis Indica in Corn Plasters and Solvents', *PJ*, 114 (1925).

'Cannabis Indica in Corn Solvents', *PJ*, 114 (1925).

'Letters to the Editor', *PJ*, 114 (1925).

'Proposed Additions to the Poison Schedule', *PJ*, 113 (1924).

RICHARDSON, B. W., 'Indian Hemp as an Intoxicant', *Abkari*, 3 (1892).

ROCHE, A., 'Symptoms of Poisoning from a Small Dose of Tincture of Cannabis Indica', *Lancet*, 2 (1898).

'Royal Medico-Botanical Society February 22 1843' *PMSJ*, 5 (1843).

SHAW, W. S. J., 'Cannabis Indica: A "Dangerous Drug"', *BMJ*, 2 (1923).

SKUES, E., 'Tetanus Treated with Extract of Indian Hemp', *EMJ*, 3 (1858).

STIRLING, A., 'Indian Hemp', *BMJ*, 2 (1897).

STRANGE, W., 'Cannabis Indica as a Medicine and as a Poison', *BMJ*, 2 (1883).

TULL WALSH, J. H., 'Hemp Drugs and Insanity', *JMS*, 40 (1894).

URQUHART, A., and TUKE, S., 'Two Visits to the Cairo Asylum, 1877 and 1878', *JMS*, 25 (1879–80).

WALLICH, G., 'Cannabis Indica', *BMJ*, 2 (1883).

WARNOCK, J., 'Twenty-Eight Years' Lunacy Experience in Egypt (1895–1923)', *JMS*, 70 (1924).

——'Insanity from Hasheesh', *JMS*, 49 (1903).

BOOKS

Historical

ACOSTA, C., *Des drogues et medicaments qui naissent aux Indes*, in A. Colin (ed.), *Histoire des drogues*.

ADAMS, H., *A Short History of Drugs etc. likewise Chinese and Lacquered Ware, the Produce of the East Indies, Published for the Sole Direction of the Commanders and Officers in that Service who are Allowed Private Trade, Homeward Bound*, (London, 1779).

AINSLIE, W., *Materia Medica of Hindoostan and Artisan's and Agriculturist's Nomenclature*, (Government Press, Madras, 1813).

——*Clemenza or The Tuscan Orphan: A Tragic Drama in Five Acts* (Cruttwell, Bath, 1822).

——*Materia Indica or some Account of those Articles which are Employed by the Hindoos and Other Eastern Nations in their Medicine, Arts and Agriculture* (Longman, Rees, Orme, Brown & Green, London, 1826).

——*An Historical Sketch of the Introduction of Christianity into India and its Progress and Present State in that and other Eastern Countries* (Oliver & Boyd, Edinburgh, 1835).

BAILEY, N., *Dictionarium Britannicum or a Compleat Universal Etymological English Dictionary* (Cox, London, 1730).

BALFOUR, J., 'Obituary Notice of Dr Greville', in *The Collected Works of Dr RK Greville on Diatomaceae* (Neill, Edinburgh, 1866).

BERLU, J., *The Treasury of Drugs Unlocked or a Full and True Description of Drugs, Chymical Preparations Sold by Druggists* (Ballard, London, 1738).

BESNARD, P., *Observations on Promoting the Cultivation of Hemp and Flax and Extending the Linen and Hempen Manufactures in the South of Ireland* (Folds, Dublin, 1816).

CAINE, W. S., *Picturesque India: A Handbook for European Travellers* (Routledge, London, 1890).

CHOPRA, R., *Chopra's Indigenous Drugs of India* (UN Dhur, Calcutta, 1958).

COLIN, A (ed.), *Histoire des drogues, espiceries et de certains medicamens simples qui naissent es Indes et en l'Amerique* (Pillehotte, Lyon, 1619).

A Concise Narrative of the Life, Travels, Collections, Works etc. of Sir Hans Sloane (Cooper, London, 1755).

COOKE, M., *The Seven Sisters of Sleep: Popular History of the Seven Prevailing Narcotics of the World* (Blackwood, London, 1860).

CROKER, T., et al., *The Complete Dictionary of Arts and Sciences in which the Whole Circle of Human Learning is Explained* (London, 1765).

The Dictionary of Trade, Commerce and Navigation (London 1844).

D'ERLANGER, H., *The Last Plague of Egypt* (Lovat Dickson & Thompson, London, 1936).

FLEMING, J., *A Catalogue of Indian Medicinal Plants and Drugs with their Names in the Hindustani and Sunscrit Languages* (Hindustani Press, Calcutta, 1810).

GREVILLE, R., 'Some Account of a Few of the More Remarkable Indian Plants in which the Species are Arranged According to the Natural Families to which they Belong', in H. Murray et al. (eds.), *Historical and Descriptive Account of British India* (Oliver & Boyd, Edinburgh, 1832).

GROSE, J., *A Voyage to the East Indies with Observations on Various Parts there* (Hooper & Morley, London, 1757).

HUDDART, J., *The Oriental Navigator or New Directions for Sailing to and from the East Indies* published with *The India Officers and Traders Guide in Purchasing the Drugs and Spices of Asia and the East Indies* (James Humphreys, Philadelphia, 1801).

IARDIN, G. DU (French spelling of G. D'Orta), *Histoire de quelques plantes des Indes*, in A. Colin (ed.), *Histoire des drogues*.

JAMES, J., and MOORE, D., *A System of Exchange with almost all Parts of the World. To which is added the India Directory* (John Furman, New York, 1800).

JAMES, R., *A Medicinal Dictionary, including Physic, Surgery, Anatomy, Chymistry and Botany in all their branches relative to medicine together with a history of drugs, an account of their various preparations, combinations, and uses* (Osborne, London, 1745).

KANE, H., *Drugs that Enslave: The Opium, Morphine, Chloral and Hashisch Habits* (Presley Blakiston, Philadelphia, 1881).

LUDLOW, F. H., *The Hasheesh-Eater* (Harper, New York, 1857).

LUNAN, J., *Hortus Jamaicensis or a Botanical Description (according to the Linnean system) and an Account of the Virtues etc. of its Indigenous Plants hitherto known as also of the most Useful Exotics Compiled from the Best Authorities and Alphabetically Arranged in Two Volumes* (St Jago de la Vega Gazette, 1814).

MARTYN, T., *The Gardener's and Botanist's Dictionary by the Late Philip Miller, The Whole Corrected and Newly Arranged* (Rivington et al., London, 1807).

MILLER, P., *The Gardener's Dictionary, Containing the Methods of Cultivating and Improving the Kitchen, Fruit and Flower Garden as also the Physick Garden, Wilderness, Conservatory and Vineyard* (Rivington, London, 1731).

MONFREID, H. DE, *Pearls, Arms and Hashish* (Gollancz, London, 1930).

——*Hashish: A Smuggler's Tale* (Penguin, London, 1946).

MOREAU, J. J., *Hashish and Mental Illness*, trans. G. Barnett (Raven Press, New York, 1973).

NEWTON, J., *W. S. Caine MP: A Biography* (Nisbet, London, 1907).

O'SHAUGHNESSY, W., *Investigation of Cases of Poisoning* (Bishops College Press, Calcutta, 1841).

——*A Manual of Chemistry Arranged for Native, General and Medical Students and the Subordinate Medical Department of the Service* (Ostell & Lepage, Calcutta, 1842).

O'SHAUGHNESSY, W., *The Bengal Dispensatory and Companion to the Pharmaco-poeia* (Allen, London, 1842).

—— *The Bengal Pharmacopoeia and General Conspectus of Medicinal Plants* (Bishops College Press, Calcutta, 1844).

ORTA, G. D', *Coloquios dos simples e drogas he cousas medicinais da India* (Ioannes Goa, 1563).

PLAYFAIR, G., *The Taleef Sereef or Indian Materia Medica (translated from the original with additions)* (Medical and Physical Society of Calcutta, 1833).

Portable Instructions for Purchasing the Drugs and Spices of Asia and the East Indies (London, 1779).

POSTLETHWAYT, M., *The Universal Dictionary of Trade and Commerce* (London, 1766).

ROLT, R., *A New Dictionary of Trade and Commerce* (London, 1756).

ROWNTREE, J., *The Opium Habit in the East: A Study of the Evidence Given to the Royal Commission on Opium 1893/4* (King, London, 1895).

ROYLE, J., *Illustrations of the Botany and other Branches of the Natural History of the Himalayan Mountains and of the Flora of Cashmere* (Allen, London, 1839).

SIMPSON, J., *The Obstetric Memoirs and Contributions of James Simpson* (Black, Edinburgh, 1855).

SLOANE, H., *A Voyage to the Islands of Madera, Barbados, Nieves, S. Christophers and Jamaica* (London, 1707).

A Subsidy granted to the king of tonnage and poundage and other sums of mony payable upon merchandize exported and imported (Bill & Barker, London, 1667).

TAYLOR, C., *Remarks on the Culture and Preparation of Hemp in Canada* (Quebec, 1806).

WATT, G., *Hemp or Cannabis Sativa (being an enlargement of the article in the 'Dictionary of Economic Products of India')* (Calcutta, 1887).

—— *A Dictionary of the Economic Products of India*, vol. ii, (Calcutta, 1889).

Who's Who in India 1911 (Newul Kishore, Lucknow, 1911).

WILLIAMS, S., *Sussex County Lunatic Asylum, Fourteenth Annual Reports for the Year 1872* (Bacon, Lewes, 1873).

WISSETT, R., *On the Cultivation and Preparation of Hemp* (Cox & Son, London, 1804).

—— *A Treatise on Hemp* (Harding, London, 1808).

YEATS, W. B., *Autobiographies* (Macmillan, London, 1926).

Contemporary

ABEL, E., *Marihuana: The First Twelve Thousand Years* (Plenum Press, London, 1980).

Academy of Medical Sciences, *The Use of Cannabis and its Derivatives for Medical and Recreational Purposes* (The Royal Society, London, 1998).

APPADURAI, A., 'Number in the Colonial Imagination', in C. A. Breckenridge and Peter van der Veer (eds.), *Orientalism and the Postcolonial Predicament: Perspectives on South Asia* (University of Pennsylvania Press, Philadelphia, 1993).

ARNOLD, D., 'The Colonial Prison: Power, Knowledge and Penology in Nine teenth-Century India' in D. Arnold and D. Hardiman (eds.), *Subaltern Studies VIII* (Oxford University Press, Oxford, 1994).

BERRIDGE, V., *Opium and the People: Opiate Use and Drug Control Policy in Nineteenth and Early Twentieth Century England* (Free Association Books, London, 1999),

——and G. EDWARDS, *Opium and the People: Opiate Use in Nineteenth Century England* (Allen Lane, London, 1981).

BONNIE, R., and WHITEBREAD, C., *The Marihuana Conviction: A History of Marihuana Prohibition in the United States* (Virginia University Press, Charlottesville, 1974).

British Medical Association, *Therapeutic Uses of Cannabis* (Harwood Academic Publishers, Amsterdam, 1997).

BOOTH, M., *Opium: A History* (Simon & Schuster, London, 1996).

BOXER, C., *Two Pioneers of Tropical Medicine: Garcia d'Orta and Nicolas Monardes* (Wellcome, London, 1963).

—— *The Dutch Seaborne Empire, 1600–1800* (Hutchinson, London, 1977).

CARDOZO, N., *Lucky Eyes and a High Heart: The Life of Maud Gonne* (Bobbs Merrill, New York, 1978).

COHN, B., 'The Census, Social Structure and Objectification in South India', in B. Cohn, *An Anthropologist among the Historians and Other Essays* (Oxford University Press, Oxford, 1987).

COURTWRIGHT, D., *Forces of Habit: Drugs and the Making of the Modern World* (Harvard University Press, London, 2001).

CRAIG, F., *British Parliamentary Election Results 1885–1918* (Macmillan, Basingstoke, 1974).

—— *British Electoral Facts 1832–1987* (Gower, Aldershot, 1989).

—— *British Parliamentary Election Results 1832–1885* (Dartmouth, Aldershot, 1989).

DALY, M., 'The British Occupation 1882–1922', in M. Daly (ed.), *The Cambridge History of Egypt*, vol. ii (Cambridge University Press, Cambridge, 1998).

EL AZHARY SONBOL, A., *The Creation of a Medical Profession in Egypt, 1800–1922* (Syracuse University Press, New York, 1991).

EMDAD-UL HAQ, M., *Drugs in South Asia: From the Opium Trade to the Present Day* (Palgrave, London, 2000).

FAHMY, K., 'The Era of Muhammad Ali Pasha', in M. Daly (ed.), *The Cambridge History of Egypt*, vol. ii (Cambridge University Press, Cambridge, 1998).

FAROOQUI, A., *Smuggling as Subversion: Colonialism, Indian Merchants and the Politics of Opium* (New Age, New Delhi, 1998).

GARDNER, J., *Yeats and the Rhymers' Club* (Lang, New York, 1989).

GOLD, M., *Cocaine* (Plenum, London, 1993)

GOURVISH, T. and WILSON, R., *The British Brewing Industry, 1830–1980* (Cambridge University Press, Cambridge, 1994).

GRINSPOON, L., *Marihuana: The Forbidden Medicine* (Yale University Press, London, 1993).

GRIVAS, K., *Cannabis, Marihuana, Hashish* trans. D. Whitehouse (Minerva Press, London, 1970).

HAINING, P. (ed.) *The Hashish Club: An Anthology of Drug Literature* (Owen, London, 1975).

HAYES, G., and SHAPIRO, H., *Drug Notes: Cannabis* (Institute for the Study of Drug Dependence, London, 1998).

HERER, J., *The Emperor Wears no Clothes: Hemp and the Marijuana Conspiracy* (Queen of Clubs Publishing, Van Nuys, Calif., 1992).

IVERSEN, L., *The Science of Marijuana* (Oxford University Press, Oxford, 2000).

JAY, M., *Emperors of Dreams: Drugs in the Nineteenth Century* (Dedalus, Sawtry, 2000).

KUHNKE, L., *Lives at Risk: Public Health in Nineteenth Century Egypt* (University of California Press, Berkeley, 1990).

LEVENSON, S., *Maud Gonne* (Cassel, London, 1976).

MCALLISTER, W., *Drug Diplomacy in the Twentieth Century* (Routledge, London, 2000).

MACK, A., and JOY, J., *Marijuana as Medicine?* (National Academy Press, Washington, 2001).

MATTHEWS, P., *Cannabis Culture: A Journey through Disputed Territory* (Bloomsbury, London, 1999).

MERLIN, M., *Man and Marijuana: Some Aspects of their Ancient Relationship* (Associated University Presses, Rutherford, NJ, 1972).

MEYER, K., and PARSSINEN, T., *Webs of Smoke* (Rowan & Littlefield, London, 1998).

MILLS, J., *Madness, Cannabis and Colonialism: The 'Native Only' Lunatic Asylums of British India, 1857 to 1900* (Macmillan, Basingstoke, 2000).

NIGAM, S., 'Disciplining and Policing the "Criminals" by Birth, Part I: The Making of a Colonial Stereotype—The Criminal Tribes of North India', *Indian Economic and Social History Review*, 27/2 (1990).

OMISSI, D., *Indian Voices of the Great War* (Macmillan, Basingstoke, 1999).

OWEN, D., *British Opium Policy in China and India* (Archon, New Heven, 1968).

ROBSON, P., *Forbidden Drugs* (Oxford University Press, Oxford, 1999).

ROSENTHAL, F., *The Herb: Hashish versus Medieval Muslim Society* (Brill, Leiden, 1971).

RUBIN, V. (ed.), *Cannabis and Culture* (Mouton, Paris, 1975).

SLOMAN, L., *The History of Marijuana in America* (Bobbs Merrill, New York, 1979).

STENTON, M., and LEES, S., *Who's Who of British Members of Parliament*, vol. ii (Harvester, Brighton, 1978).

TAYLOR, A., *American Diplomacy and the Narcotics Traffic 1900–1939* (Duke University Press, Durham, NC, 1969).

TOIT, BRIAN DU, 'Dagga: The History and Ethnographic Setting of Cannabis Sativa in Southern Africa', in Rubin, *Cannabis and Culture*.

TOLEN, R., 'Colonizing and Transforming the Criminal Tribesman: The Salvation Army in British India', in J. Urla and J. Terry (eds.), *Deviant Bodies: Critical Perspectives on Difference in Science and Popular Culture* (Indiana University Press, Bloomington, 1995).

TROCKI, C., *Opium, Empire and the Global Political Economy* (Routledge, London, 1999).

WALKER, W., *Opium and Foreign Policy: The Anglo-American Search for Order in Asia, 1912–1954* (University of North Carolina Press, Durham, NC, 1991).

——*Drugs in the Western Hemisphere* (Scholarly Resources, Wilmington, 1996).

WALTON, S., *Out of It: A Cultural History of Intoxication* (Hamish Hamilton, London, 2001).

Index